ALTERNATIVES TO
THE HOSPITAL FOR ACUTE
PSYCHIATRIC TREATMENT

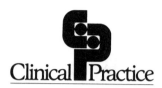

Clinical Practice

Number 32

Judith H. Gold, M.D., F.R.C.P.C.
Series Editor

ALTERNATIVES TO THE HOSPITAL FOR ACUTE PSYCHIATRIC TREATMENT

Edited by

Richard Warner, M.B., D.P.M.

Medical Director, Mental Health Center of Boulder County
Associate Clinical Professor, Department of Psychiatry
Associate Professor–Adjunct, Department of Anthropology
University of Colorado

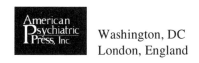

Washington, DC
London, England

American Psychiatric Press, Inc.
1400 K Street, N.W., Washington, DC 20005

Library of Congress Cataloging-in-Publication Data
Alternatives to the hospital for acute psychiatric treatment / edited
    by Richard Warner. — 1st ed.
        p.   cm. — (Clinical practice ; no. 32)
    Includes bibliographical references and index.
    ISBN 0-88048-484-5
    1. Alternatives to psychiatric hospitalization.   I. Warner,
Richard, 1943-   . II. Series.
    [DNLM: 1. Mental Health Services—organization & administration.
    2. Health Facilities—organization & administration.   3. Home Care
Services—organization & administration.   W1 CL767J no.32 1995 / WM
30 A4663   1995]
RC439.7.A46   1995
362.2—dc20
DNLM/DLC
for Library of Congress   95-34
                                                                       CIP

British Library Cataloguing in Publication Data
A CIP record is available from the British Library.

Contents

Contributors

Elisabeth Aebi, lic. phil.
Psychologist, Socio-Psychiatric University Clinic, Berne, Switzerland

Russell Bennett, R.N.
Manager, Family Crisis Homes, Dane County Mental Center, Madison, Wisconsin

Pauline Bourgeois, M.S.W., Ph.D.
Director, Crossing Place, Washington, DC

Luc Ciompi, M.D.
Professor of Psychiatry and Medical Director, Socio-Psychiatric University Clinic, Berne, Switzerland

Hans-Peter Dauwalder, Ph.D.
Professor of Psychology, Socio-Psychiatric University Clinic, Berne, Switzerland

Walter S. Deitchman, M.S.W.
former Project Coordinator, Colorado Community Support Project at Southwest Denver Community Mental Health Services, Denver, Colorado, and currently Health Service Consultant in Denver, Colorado

Daniel Dowd
former Program Director, Northwest Evaluation and Treatment Center, Seattle, Washington

William D. Ferguson, M.D.
Staff Psychiatrist, Northwest Evaluation and Treatment Center, Seattle, Washington

Steven L. Fields, M.P.A.
Director, Progress Foundation, San Francisco, California

Jeffrey M. Fortuna, M.A.
Director, Windhorse Associates, Inc., Northampton, Massachusetts

David B. Goldblatt, M.A.
Director, Burch House, Inc., Littleton, New Hampshire

Rollande Hamilton, R.P.N.
Unit Manager, Venture, Greater Vancouver Mental Health Service
Society, Vancouver, British Columbia

Michael W. Kirby, Ph.D.
former Director of Research and Evaluation, Southwest Denver
Community Mental Health Services, and currently Executive
Director, Arapahoe House, Denver, Colorado

Zeno Kupper, Ph.D.
Psychologist, Socio-Psychiatric University Clinic, Berne, Switzerland

Christian Maier, M.D.
Psychiatrist, Socio-Psychiatric University Clinic, Berne, Switzerland

James Mandiberg, L.C.S.W.
former Director, Community Mental Health Services for Santa Clara
County, California, former Associate Professor, Department of
Social Welfare, Shikoku Gakuin University, Zentsuji, Japan, and
currently completing his doctorate in social work and organizational
psychology at the University of Michigan, Ann Arbor

Loren R. Mosher, M.D.
Associate Director, Montgomery County Department of Addiction,
Victim and Mental Health Services, Rockville, Maryland; Clinical
Professor of Psychiatry, Uniformed Services University of the Health
Sciences, Bethesda, Maryland

Hugh Parfitt, M.B., F.R.C.P.C.
Medical Director, Greater Vancouver Mental Health Service Society,
Vancouver, British Columbia

Paul R. Polak, M.D.
former Executive Director, Southwest Denver Community Mental
Health Services, Denver, Colorado, and currently Executive Director
of International Development Enterprises, Lakewood, Colorado

Charlotte Rutishauser, lic. phil.
Psychologist, Socio-Psychiatric University Clinic, Berne, Switzerland

Willem J. Schudel, M.D., Ph.D.
Professor and Chairman, Department of Psychiatry, Dijkzigt
Hospital, Erasmus University, Rotterdam, the Netherlands

Nicholas Sladen-Dew, M.B., Ch.B., M.P.H., F.R.C.P.C.
Associate Medical Director, Greater Vancouver Mental Health
Service Society, Vancouver, British Columbia

Karl Trütsch, M.D.
Psychiatrist, Socio-Psychiatric University Clinic, Berne, Switzerland

Richard Warner, M.B., D.P.M.
Medical Director, Mental Health Center of Boulder County, Boulder,
Colorado; Associate Clinical Professor, Department of Psychiatry
and Associate Professor–Adjunct, Department of Anthropology,
University of Colorado

Charlotte Wollesen, M.A.
Team Leader, Inpatient Services, Mental Health Center of Boulder
County, Boulder, Colorado

Anne-Marie Young, R.N.
Assistant Unit Manager, Venture, Greater Vancouver Mental Health
Service Society, Vancouver, British Columbia

Introduction
to the Clinical Practice Series

Over the years of its existence the series of monographs entitled *Clinical Insights* gradually became focused on providing current, factual, and theoretical material of interest to the clinician working outside of a hospital setting. To reflect this orientation, the name of the Series has been changed to *Clinical Practice.*

The Clinical Practice Series will provide books that give the mental health clinician a practical, clinical approach to a variety of psychiatric problems. These books will provide up-to-date literature reviews and emphasize the most recent treatment methods. Thus, the publications in the Series will interest clinicians working both in psychiatry and in the other mental health professions.

Each year a number of books will be published dealing with all aspects of clinical practice. In addition, from time to time when appropriate, the publications may be revised and updated. Thus, the Series will provide quick access to relevant and important areas of psychiatric practice. Some books in the Series will be authored by a person considered to be an expert in that particular area; others will be edited by such an expert, who will also draw together other knowledgeable authors to produce a comprehensive overview of that topic.

This particular book on alternatives to acute psychiatric hospitalization is somewhat different from most of the previous and future editions of the books in this Series. The authors of the various chapters discuss alternatives to the usual care offered to acutely ill psychiatric patients. Many of their programs are unique. Most have not had the standard form of scientific evaluation to which we are accustomed. However, they all have been described by the authors in some detail, and the benefits that these professionals find the alternatives offer for their patients are presented for your information. I encourage you to make your own decisions about alternative types of care and to make your own evaluation. I hope that you will find this book to be interesting and thought challenging.

Some of the books in the Clinical Practice Series will have their foundation in presentations at an annual meeting of the American Psychiatric Association. All will contain the most recently available information on the subjects discussed. Theoretical and scientific data will be applied to clinical situations, and case illustrations will be utilized in order to make the material even more relevant for the practitioner. Thus, the Clinical Practice Series should provide educational reading in a compact format especially designed for the mental health clinician–psychiatrist.

Judith H. Gold, M.D., F.R.C.P.C.
Series Editor
Clinical Practice Series

Clinical Practice Series Titles

Alternatives to the Hospital for Acute Psychiatric Treatment (#32)
Edited by Richard Warner, M.B., D.P.M.

Behavioral Complications in Alzheimer's Disease (#31)
Edited by Brian A. Lawlor, M.D.

Clinician Safety (#30)
Edited by Burr Eichelman, M.D., Ph.D.

Effective Use of Group Therapy in Managed Care (#29)
Edited by K. Roy MacKenzie, M.D., F.R.C.P.C.

Rediscovering Childhood Trauma: Historical Casebook and Clinical Applications (#28)
Edited by Jean M. Goodwin, M.D., M.P.H.

Treatment of Adult Survivors of Incest (#27)
Edited by Patricia L. Paddison, M.D.

Madness and Loss of Motherhood: Sexuality, Reproduction, and Long-Term Mental Illness (#26)
Edited by Roberta J. Apfel, M.D., M.P.H., and Maryellen H. Handel, Ph.D.

Psychiatric Aspects of Symptom Management in Cancer Patients (#25)
Edited by William Breitbart, M.D., and Jimmie C. Holland, M.D.

Responding to Disaster: A Guide for Mental Health Professionals (#24)
Edited by Linda S. Austin, M.D.

Psychopharmacological Treatment Complications in the Elderly (#23)
Edited by Charles A. Shamoian, M.D., Ph.D.

Anxiety Disorders in Children and Adolescents (#22)
By Syed Arshad Husain, M.D., F.R.C.P.C., F.R.C.Psych., and
Javad Kashani, M.D.

Suicide and Clinical Practice (#21)
Edited by Douglas Jacobs, M.D.

Special Problems in Managing Eating Disorders (#20)
Edited by Joel Yager, M.D., Harry E. Gwirtsman, M.D., and
Carole K. Edelstein, M.D.

Children and AIDS (#19)
Edited by Margaret L. Stuber, M.D.

Current Treatments of Obsessive-Compulsive Disorder (#18)
Edited by Michele Tortora Pato, M.D., and Joseph Zohar, M.D.

Benzodiazepines in Clinical Practice: Risks and Benefits (#17)
Edited by Peter P. Roy-Byrne, M.D., and Deborah S. Cowley, M.D.

Adolescent Psychotherapy (#16)
Edited by Marcia Slomowitz, M.D.

Family Approaches in Treatment of Eating Disorders (#15)
Edited by D. Blake Woodside, M.D., M.Sc., F.R.C.P.C.,and
Lorie Shekter-Wolfson, M.S.W., C.S.W.

**Clinical Management of Gender Identity Disorders in
Children and Adults (#14)**
Edited by Ray Blanchard, Ph.D., and Betty W. Steiner, M.B., F.R.C.P.C.

New Perspectives on Narcissism (#13)
Edited by Eric M. Plakun, M.D.

The Psychosocial Impact of Job Loss (#12)
By Nick Kates, M.B.B.S., F.R.C.P.C., Barrie S. Greiff, M.D., and
Duane Q. Hagen, M.D.

Office Treatment of Schizophrenia (#11)
Edited by Mary V. Seeman, M.D., F.R.C.P.C., and
Stanley E. Greben, M.D., F.R.C.P.C.

Psychiatric Care of Migrants: A Clinical Guide (#10)
By Joseph Westermeyer, M.D., M.P.H., Ph.D.

Family Involvement in Treatment of the Frail Elderly (#9)
Edited by Marion Zucker Goldstein, M.D.

**Measuring Mental Illness: Psychometric Assessment
for Clinicians (#8)**
Edited by Scott Wetzler, Ph.D.

Juvenile Homicide (#7)
Edited by Elissa P. Benedek, M.D., and Dewey G. Cornell, Ph.D.

The Neuroleptic Malignant Syndrome and Related Conditions (#6)
By Arthur Lazarus, M.D., Stephan C. Mann, M.D., and
Stanley N. Caroff, M.D.

Anxiety: New Findings for the Clinician (#5)
Edited by Peter Roy-Byrne, M.D.

Anxiety and Depressive Disorders in the Medical Patient (#4)
By Leonard R. Derogatis, Ph.D., and Thomas N. Wise, M.D.

Family Violence: Emerging Issues of a National Crisis (#3)
Edited by Leah J. Dickstein, M.D., and Carol C. Nadelson, M.D.

Divorce as a Developmental Process (#2)
Edited by Judith H. Gold, M.D., F.R.C.P.C.

Treating Chronically Mentally Ill Women (#1)
Edited by Leona L. Bachrach, Ph.D., and Carol C. Nadelson, M.D.

Introduction

Richard Warner, M.B., D.P.M.

*D*omestic settings for the treatment of adult acutely disturbed, mentally ill patients offer a number of benefits. They provide care that is more cost-effective, less coercive, and less alienating than hospital treatment. Despite these advantages, there are fewer such treatment settings in the United States than might be expected, considering the number of patients who can benefit.

In this volume, a range of acute nonhospital treatment programs from the United States and abroad are described—locked and open-door settings, voluntary and involuntary, public and private, and nontraditional and strictly medical. Details of staffing, management, and cost are provided. The program descriptions make it clear which types of patients can and cannot be treated successfully in the various settings and how these programs function within the broader mental health system.

Why are there not more such programs in the United States? Current health insurance mechanisms do not support their use. Managed care providers are becoming aware, however, that nonhospital programs offer substantial cost-benefit advantages. In Boulder, Colorado, for example, a number of health maintenance organizations now contract with the community mental health center for emergency psychiatric and inpatient services, in part because the range of inpatient options offered by the center includes a hospital alternative (described in Chapter 1) that costs one-quarter of psychiatric hospital care. Where Medicaid capitation schemes for the provision of health care are being introduced—for instance, in Utah and Colorado—we can expect to see hospital-alternative settings, with their opportunities for cost saving, become used more frequently in preference to conventional care.

Sufficient details are provided throughout the book for mental health administrators to evaluate the usefulness and feasibility of the various models for their own communities and systems of care and for clinicians, patients, and their families to understand what it is like to live or work in one of these treatment environments. The reader will understand how a hospital alternative can provide a truly alternative style of treatment, not just the usual care in a different setting.

Case examples and self-reports from the customer's point of view are used to illustrate how different these settings are and why they produce a different result. People receiving services in a noninstitutional setting are called on to use their own inner resources. They must exercise a degree of self-control and accept responsibility for their actions and for the preservation of their living environment. Consequently, patients retain more of their self-respect, their skills, and their sense of mastery. The domestic and noncoercive nature of the alternatives described in this book makes human contact with the person in crisis easier than it is in hospitals. As Steve Fields writes of psychiatric hospitals in Chapter 4 on the Progress Foundation,

> We take our most frightened, most alienated, and most confused patients and place them in environments that increase fear, alienation, and confusion . . . we practice our trade in settings that are toxic to relationships and human interaction.

There are common origins for many of these alternative settings for the treatment of acute mental disorders. Some (e.g., Paul Polak's innovative program described in Chapter 12) have links to the postwar therapeutic community movement, of which British psychiatrist Maxwell Jones was a major force. Others (Soteria and Burch House in Chapters 7 and 9, respectively) trace their roots back to the experimental treatment environments of R. D. Laing and his associates in the Philadelphia Association in London in the 1960s. A series of programs in the Netherlands, described in Chapter 6, was developed in response to the concept of primary prevention of emotional disorder espoused by Gerald Caplan in his 1963 book, *The Principles of Preventive Psychiatry.*

The thread runs back through these revolutionary postwar developments in social psychiatry to an even earlier source—to the successful elements of early nineteenth-century moral management. There are common themes—active ingredients—in these alternative treatment programs and the models, from this century and the last, to which they are linked, which tell us something about the human needs of patients and the nature of the illnesses being treated. Now, as in the moral treatment era, effective psychosocial treatment settings tend to be small, family-style, and normalizing. They are open-door, genuinely in the community, and allow the user to stay in touch with his or her friends, relatives, work, and social life. They are flexible and noncoercive and are often based more on peer relationships than on hierarchical power structures. They involve residents in running their own environment and use whatever work capacity the patient has to offer. The pace of treatment is not as fast as in a hospital, and the units generally try to provide a quiet form of genuine "asylum."

The success of these treatment strategies suggests ways in which we should be redesigning hospital care and rebuilding treatment systems. The reader can draw general conclusions about the humane care of mentally ill patients—about the value of role blurring and the importance of empowering the patient and engaging him or her in the process of recovery, about the insidious effects of alienation, and the necessity for the patient to develop a sense of self-control. These observations are valuable to mental health professionals working in a broad variety of treatment settings—much broader than the alternative settings described in this book.

Some of the programs, for example, Cedar House in Colorado (Chapter 1), Venture in British Columbia (Chapter 2), and the crisis intervention centers in the Netherlands (Chapter 6), have been functioning as integral elements of established treatment systems since the 1970s. Others, such as Burch House in New Hampshire (Chapter 9) and the Buddhist-influenced Windhorse program in Massachusetts (Chapter 10), are independent and assertively unconventional in nature. All of the programs described in this book, however, are somewhat nontraditional and, except in the case of the California-based Soteria project (Chapter 7) and Soteria-Berne in Switzerland (Chapter 8), have not been evaluated by rigorous comparative research. The programs have worked well in the hands of their creators and current operators, but readers will recognize that to establish a similar program in a new context requires prudent evaluation, planning, and possible modifications of the model.

Part I

Programs in the Mainstream

Editor's Note

CEDAR HOUSE WAS DEVELOPED 15 YEARS AGO AS A PROGRAM OF A comprehensive community mental health center to control ballooning inpatient costs. Inpatient treatment at Cedar House costs one-quarter of the daily rate in local psychiatric hospital wards. The program is not only less expensive; it has proved its worth in a number of other ways. Patients and staff prefer Cedar House because it is less confining, noncoercive, and nonalienating. The emphasis on individual self-control means that severely disturbed patients behave less aggressively at Cedar House than they would in a hospital. The important features of the program are that it is fairly small, domestic in style although assertively medical in treatment orientation, and more attractive to patients than hospitals, so that they make an effort to comply with the rules of the household.

Two cases are described to illustrate the range of disorders successfully treated in this setting, and comparisons can be made with hospital treatment. The treatment experience of one patient is recounted by his father; in the second case, the patient describes her own reactions to Cedar House.

Cedar House: A Noncoercive Hospital Alternative in Boulder, Colorado

Richard Warner, M.B., D.P.M.
Charlotte Wollesen, M.A., and others*

Cedar House is a large house on a busy residential street in Boulder, Colorado (Figure 1–1). Staffed, as one would staff an acute psychiatric hospital ward, with nurses, a psychiatrist, and mental health workers, it functions as an alternative to the psychiatric hospital for the acutely disturbed patients of the Mental Health Center of Boulder County. Like a hospital, it offers all the usual diagnostic and treatment services (except electroconvulsive therapy [ECT]). Routine medical evaluations are performed on the premises: patients requiring advanced medical and neurological investigation, including those with acute or chronic organic brain disorders, are evaluated by consulting physicians and in local hospital departments. Unlike a hospital, it is homelike, unlocked, and noncoercive.

As much as possible, Cedar House has the appearance of a middle-class home, not a hospital. Residents and staff may bring their pets with them to the house. A bird can be heard singing in one of the bedrooms, and a dog shares the comfortable furniture with the residents. On winter nights, a fire burns in the hearth. Staff and patients interact casually and share household duties. Residents come and go fairly freely (some attend work while in treatment), when they have negotiated passes with the therapist. Staff must encourage patients to comply willingly with treatment and house rules: no one can be strapped down, locked in, or

---

* This chapter was written in collaboration with consumer authors whose names are withheld to protect confidentiality.

medicated by force. Many patients, nevertheless, are treated involuntarily at Cedar House under the provisions of the state mental illness

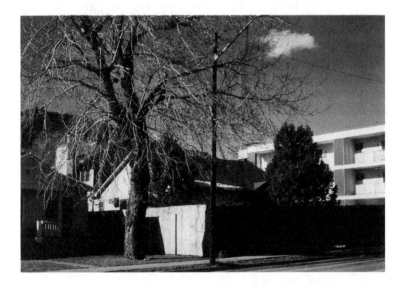

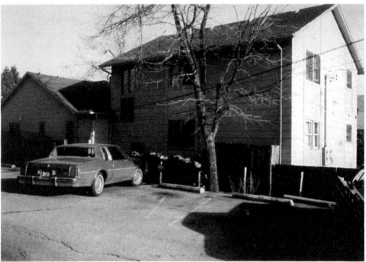

Figure 1–1.   Cedar House, Boulder, Colorado.

statute; they accept the restrictions because the alternative is hospital treatment, which virtually none prefer.

The Patients

People who are violent or threatening, who repeatedly walk away, who are so loud and agitated that they would make the house intolerable for other residents, or who are so confused that they cannot follow staff direction cannot be treated in the house. In practice, almost every person with a psychotic depression, most people with an acute episode of schizophrenia, and many people with mania can be treated in the facility. Very few patients (fewer than 10%) need to be transferred to the hospital. Cedar House has not entirely replaced locked hospital care, but it provides nearly two-thirds of the acute inpatient treatment for the mental health center's patients and could provide an even greater proportion if more beds of this type were available.

Most patients needing admission have symptoms of psychosis or affective disorder, but those with adjustment disorders or personality disorders are sometimes appropriate for admission. Many patients have a dual diagnosis of mental illness with substance abuse, and some have mental illness with intellectual impairment.

The following types of patients would be more likely to be admitted to a hospital than to Cedar House:

- Patients who are likely to elope from Cedar House and who, as a result, would be very likely to suffer significantly (e.g., those with serious suicide risk or gravely disabled and confused patients)
- Patients who pose a significant risk of hurting themselves or someone else or of damaging property (e.g., people who have shown recent random violence)
- Extremely agitated and noncompliant people (this is likely to apply to severely disturbed manic patients)
- Patients who have direct access to guns and who present some risk of using them

Issues that definitely *don't*, by themselves, preclude admission to Cedar House include

- Severe psychosis.
- Concurrent medical problems.

- Organic brain pathology.
- Suicidal ideas or gestures.
- Age—any age above 16 is acceptable; people over age 65 are commonly admitted.
- Social class—although it sometimes takes a while for new upper-middle-class patients and their families to perceive the advantages that Cedar House may have over a private hospital setting (see the case examples, below).
- Ability to pay for treatment—those who have good hospital insurance are no more likely to be admitted to the hospital and those with no insurance are not rejected for Cedar House; care is provided under the center's usual sliding scale and some patients contribute toward their board and rent.
- Unpleasant disposition.
- Crabs, infectious hepatitis, acquired immunodeficiency syndrome (AIDS), or any contagious conditions that can be controlled by standard infectious precautions.

Treatment

As both cases presented later in this chapter illustrate, it has become apparent that a number of the people treated in Cedar House would be subject to coercive measures, such as restraints and seclusion, if they were admitted to a hospital where such approaches are available and routinely used. The avoidance of coercion is an important benefit of the residential program—important in maintaining the mentally ill person's sense of self-esteem and self-control. As the moral treatment advocates of the early nineteenth century discovered, treating people with respect in a homelike and normalizing environment leads them to exercise "moral restraint," or self-control over their impulses. In someone's home, one feels obliged to treat other people and property with a degree of consideration, but in an institution, anything goes.

The normalizing treatment style has many of the features of the therapeutic community approach. Residents take a hand in the day-to-day operations of the household. Every patient has a daily chore, and one resident—the chore-leader—supervises the work of others. Higher-functioning residents assist in aspects of treatment and may, for example, escort the more disturbed patients on trips outside the house when needed. Although the engagement of patients in the management of the household and in the treatment process is empowering, the extent of patient government is limited. This is because of the brief length of patient stay and the necessity for staff to exercise close control over admissions and discharges, to make room available at all times for new admissions.

Cedar House is busy. Patients are admitted at any hour of the day or night, as in a hospital. All new patients go through a formal admission procedure and are seen by a psychiatrist within 24 hours. There are usually about 20 to 25 admissions per month. The need to create bed vacancies for the next emergency admission places pressure on staff and patients alike to limit length of stay to a brief efficient period. Most patients stay a week or two but some stay much longer. The occasional person who stays months is generally a high-risk patient, sometimes potentially dangerous, sometimes medically unstable, who proves difficult to place in the community even with extensive supports and elaborate treatment.

An essential initial step in the treatment of those entering Cedar House is the evaluation of the client's social system. What has happened to bring the person in at this point in time? What are his or her financial circumstances, living arrangements, and employment status? Have there been recent changes? Are there family tensions? Has the person relapsed more since establishing the current living arrangements? From the answers to such questions, a short- and long-term treatment plan is developed. It is hoped that this plan will lead to the patient's immediate improvement, as well as reduce the chances of relapse after discharge. The goal for all patients is to leave Cedar House for suitable living conditions and coordinated treatment designed to prevent the revolving-door syndrome and to provide a decent quality of life. Virtually no one who leaves is expected to stay at a homeless shelter.

A distinct advantage of intensive residential treatment over hospital care is that the lower cost allows treatment to proceed at a more leisurely pace. More time can be spent observing the features and course of the patient's illness, selecting and adjusting medications, eliminating side effects, and evaluating benefits of treatment. Selected patients with psychoses with a good prognosis can be treated without recourse to antipsychotic drugs. Cedar House, it is true, is more institutional than some community-based alternatives, such as intensive in-home treatment of acutely disturbed psychotic patients provided by mobile teams (Brook et al. 1976). It has the advantage, however, of relying less heavily on rapid tranquilization and heavy doses of the antipsychotic drugs than is common in some in-home treatment programs.

Benzodiazepines are used extensively at Cedar House as a supplement, or sometimes as an alternative, to the antipsychotic drugs. Moderate doses of benzodiazepines, such as diazepam or lorazepam, have been found to be more effective than neuroleptics in calming acutely agitated and psychotic patients and have proven to be invaluable in the early phases of treatment in Cedar House's open-door setting. Newly admitted patients with psychotic relapse are routinely treated with modest maintenance doses of neuroleptic medication combined with flexible, as needed, doses of a benzodiazepine.

Safety is a very important issue for patients and staff, and every effort is made to ensure that no one becomes aggressive. Crisis intervention techniques are used to de-escalate arguments or acute upsets, and the staff pays careful attention to any patients who have concerns about someone becoming dangerous. Agitated patients may be offered medication or hospitalized if necessary. The staff works as a team, and each person has the opportunity and the responsibility to give input into the treatment along with the therapist and the client. This helps everyone involved have an investment in the success of the admission to Cedar House. Because the expectation at Cedar House is that people are safe and harm to others is not tolerated, everyone is expected to treat everyone else with respect. Patients are generally supportive of one another and, along with staff, are culture carriers for nonviolence and safety.

Staffing

Residential treatment of this intensity requires a staffing pattern similar to that of a hospital. A mental health worker (psychiatric aide) and a nurse are on duty at all times. On weekdays, two experienced therapists with psychology or social work degrees provide services to the residents; they offer psychotherapy, family therapy, and help with practical issues like obtaining disability benefits, and they make arrangements for the client's move back to the community. A half-time consumer case manager aide—a person who has experienced serious mental illness and has been trained in the principles of case management—also assists residents with practical issues of accommodation and entitlements. A psychiatrist is present for 3 hours a day, and an on-call psychiatrist is available by telephone around the clock. A team leader directs the program, and a secretarial assistant manages the office work, building repairs, and purchasing of supplies, food, and furnishings. Students and volunteers provide help in various ways.

A part-time cook prepares the meals with help from the mental health worker. In the early days of Cedar House, the residents did much of the cooking, but complaints were so plentiful that this is now rare. A cleaning person comes in a few times a week. Many of the patients are too dysfunctional to assist much in the upkeep of the house, cooking, or repairs, and the staff members are too busy doing other things. The house is cleaner, the food is of better quality, and things work better if these extras are squeezed into the budget.

Cedar House is staffed by people with diverse backgrounds and skills who are experienced in the care and treatment of severely mentally ill patients. For the sake of quality of care, morale, and safety, it is important to have at least two staff members in the house at all times, and because of the severity and acuity of the illnesses, it is also necessary for one of the staff on duty to be a nurse. On the night shift, the nurse sleeps, but is available if needed.

Selection of staff is important. Individuals must have high professional standards, be bright and flexible, and be able to handle crisis situations and work under stress. Staff members must be positive, friendly, and able to work well with other people. They must also genuinely enjoy working with the patients and must treat people with respect and dignity.

Supervision and communication are critical to the effective operation of the household. It is important that each staff member receive supervision on a regular basis. The work is draining and often involves taking some risks. Therapists and shift workers need to feel that they have someone with whom they can consult and who will be supportive of their efforts. The team leader provides formal supervision of the nursing coordinator, the office manager, the therapists, and the head mental health worker and is available and visible as a stabilizing influence to all staff. The psychiatrist must believe in the noncoercive treatment model and be willing to trust the staff and patients to make it work.

High morale comes from the feeling of doing a good job and

having positive interactions with others—patients and staff alike. It is important to maintain a pleasant, noncoercive atmosphere in which all play a part and feel that their contribution is important.

Management Issues

It has turned out to be important that Cedar House was set up in a neighborhood that is partly commercial. Patients can use the many nearby community resources. Within half a block are grocery stores, a drug store, a satellite post office, a coffee shop, and a general hospital emergency room. Only a few blocks away are a large park and a recreation center. Over the years, neighbors have expressed little concern. Early on it was necessary to erect a privacy fence around the property, and measures are taken to keep the noise down, especially at night, but for the most part, there are very few complaints.

The required level of staffing at Cedar House imposes relatively high fixed costs that cannot be reduced without significantly altering the nature of the program. The therapeutic design would be improved if there were fewer than 15 acutely disturbed patients in residence, but this can only be achieved by driving up the per capita daily cost or by reducing staffing to a level that would restrict the severity of illness of the patients who can be treated.

At $140 a day, Cedar House costs less than one-quarter as much as private hospital treatment. Only a small proportion of the actual costs, however, are covered by reimbursement from the patient or insurance companies. The program is not considered a hospital, and so most insurance companies will not reimburse the treatment at an inpatient rate: Medicaid pays for the treatment at the long-partial-care rate. Some health maintenance organizations (HMOs), however, appreciate that Cedar House is a bargain when the alternative is expensive hospital care and have begun to reimburse the mental health center for Cedar House treatment at the full rate. When capitated Medicaid mental health reimbursement mechanisms are established in Colorado (which may be soon), contracting mental health agencies will find inexpensive nonhospital settings like Cedar House to be far more attractive than traditional hospital units. Until then, the real reason that Cedar House is financially viable is that it offers a treatment alternative for acutely ill patients who have no medical insurance at all: a small number of such patients being treated in hospital at a daily rate of more than $600 would cost the mental health center a substantial amount of money.

The high fixed costs of Cedar House would be difficult to justify for a mental health agency with a catchment area much below 200,000. With this proviso, the Cedar House model is appropriate for both rural and urban settings. The Colorado Division of Mental Health recently replicated the Cedar House design in the northern part of the state and on the western slope of the Rockies as closer-to-home alternatives to state hospital admission for rural areas.

Case Examples

The following cases illustrate some of the differences between Cedar House and a traditional inpatient setting, the type of patients who can be treated, and some of the advantages of the program.

Case 1

The first case account is written by the father of a patient who was treated at Cedar House for a psychosis with severe catatonic features.

> Our son was a good student and, prior to college, quite active in extracurricular activities including music, theater, dance, and choir. His summers were filled with bike racing and associated activities. He was popular, quite active socially, and had several girlfriends. He was and is a sensitive and sincere person.
>
> He attended a university in Colorado, except during his sophomore year when he studied theater in New York. He graduated with a degree in humanities. The first noticeable personality changes occurred during the year he spent in New York. His sister, who was employed in the area, observed episodes of depression. Later he began psychotherapy, which continued on and off until graduation, when he returned to our home in Colorado. As part of his therapy he began to meditate to relieve anxiety. After a year, however, he was in meditation up to 50% of his waking life, and then these periods extended into the night; it became clear that he could not stop. Early one morning at about 4 A.M. I awoke and, making my way through the house, was startled by a figure standing in the middle of the family room. It was our son standing upright and motionless with dilated pupils. Blood had pooled in his extremities, leaving his hands and feet purple and somewhat swollen.
>
> He was admitted voluntarily to a private psychiatric hospital and

agreed to a small dose of medication, which had a minimal effect. In the hospital he moved so slowly that it was not possible for him to maintain his personal hygiene. The hospital did not help with this, and on occasion I assisted him in the shower. The hospital did not seem to be oriented toward treating severely ill people but rather focused on patients who were less impaired. Our son was in the hospital for about 6 weeks and was discharged shortly before his insurance benefits expired. His condition had deteriorated during his 6-week hospital stay. Although he had walked into the hospital, he required a wheelchair to leave and return home.

At home his condition continued to deteriorate. Eating or showering would take hours. His stupor increased, but he could respond by shaking his head "yes" or "no" in response to questions. He continued to slow until he could not eat or drink, and, after 2 days, an ambulance was called and he was taken to a community hospital where he was given intravenous fluids. Five days later he was discharged to home.

At home, he did manage to eat, but it became an all-day event. For example, it would be dinner time by the time lunch was finished and dinner would be completed as late as 11 P.M. On days when he showered he could not eat, because a shower would take 6 to 8 hours: water was kept at a trickle so as to remain warm. He became constipated and his bowel movements were accompanied by blood. It was impossible to provide adequate care at home, and it seemed unlikely that the private psychiatric hospital would help. Insurance benefits for the year had expired, so we approached the mental health center, and our son was admitted to Cedar House.

The accommodations at Cedar House are somewhat spartan compared with the psychiatric hospital, but there is 24-hour medical attention and therapy on a daily basis. Our son agreed to take diazepam (Valium), and after a week his condition had slightly improved. He was very thin (138 pounds) but began drinking nutritional supplements provided by the staff. He refused any other medication, and a court date was set to determine if medications could be administered to him involuntarily.

At the hearing, the judge ruled against involuntary administration of medication. Back at Cedar House, however, our son's condition deteriorated following his courtroom appearance. He remained in bed, essentially mute. He was transferred to the community hospital because he had stopped eating and had developed a urinary tract infection. A second court date was scheduled approximately 1 week after the first date. Several doctors testified that his life was at risk, and I testified that my son's last words could very well be "I will take no medications." The judge reversed his ruling and ordered that involuntary medications be administered.

He remained at Cedar House for almost 8 months, taking medications and showing gradual improvement. One of the most important advantages of Cedar House versus the private psychiatric hospital is the luxury to improve at a slow rate. The clock ticks very loudly at the psychiatric hospital; this, in itself, can create stress in the environment that is not conducive to a healing process. Cedar House provided a safe refuge where our son could improve at his own pace.

The psychiatrist and treatment team reviewed our son's progress daily, the therapist provided daily psychotherapy, and a volunteer visited every week to take him on activities, such as movies, hiking, and snacks in the local cafés, and to engage him in conversation to bring him out of his thought world. Weekly visits to a physical therapist helped to improve his posture, neck pain, and muscle stiffness.

After 8 months, our son still moved at a rate that was about one-half to one-quarter of normal. His psychiatrist recommended ECT, which he refused. The staff continued to talk to him about ECT, however, and drove him to Denver to talk with a psychiatrist at the university hospital about it. Shortly thereafter he agreed to ECT, was admitted to the hospital, and received nine treatments. The response was dramatic! He became much more communicative and regained his sense of humor. He talked more and showed his emotions normally. We told our relatives that our son was back! Unfortunately, the improvement was short-lived. Slowing was soon evident, and, within 10 days of discharge from the hospital, the situation was critical and our son was once again admitted to Cedar House. He refused further ECT but accepted medications. A new antidepressant was started, and he continued to improve.

Over the past 2 years we have followed our son's care in a private psychiatric hospital, a psychiatric ward of a general hospital, a university psychiatric hospital, and Cedar House. Although Cedar House lacks the "glitz" of the private facility, it has the feeling of home. It is an unlocked household whose members contribute to its upkeep through the assignment of chores. The importance of the Cedar House approach to the care of its patients was simply not evident to us when we first interviewed the staff and viewed the facilities. Indeed, we chose to provide our son with the "glitz" associated with the private facility, which, as we determined later, was a mistake.

After about 3 months in the private facility, we were, in fact, forced by financial realities to make use of Cedar House. At that point it was looking much more "glitzy" because our son was very ill and we had no other recourse. We believe that Cedar House was literally a lifesaver for our son. If the money had been there, would our son have been better off at the private facility? For us the answer is simple. Our son improved at Cedar House, and, moreover, he has repeatedly told us that he prefers the homelike feeling of Cedar House over the other facilities.

From our view as parents, some of the things that seem to make Cedar House work are the psychiatric leadership and the links to other treatment programs. For example, Cedar House has access to other mental health center facilities such as the clubhouse and the sheltered workshop and good working relationships with the county attorney.

Psychiatric wards feel quite different from Cedar House. Cedar House seems like a relatively normal household, whereas the hospital treats a wide range of patients, including those requiring restraints. These patients can be seen by a passing glance through small square windows, and at times they can be heard on the ward. The fact that they are in isolation does not seem to lessen the impact on those who are less ill. This creates an atmosphere of anxiety and agitation among the patients. The environment is a key factor in healing the mind. Perhaps the psychiatric ward is not the best place for some individuals.

In the hospital, patients and staff are physically separated by the traditional nursing station—a constant reminder that the patient is ill (relative to the staff). The Cedar House environment is closer to normal and, as such, motivates a wellness psychology and minimizes the adjustment required by the patient on discharge.

Cedar House is sought after by patients in the hospital because of its normal household environment. Hence, the thought of discharge from Cedar House to a psychiatric ward is a significant deterrent to harmful acts. Our son reports that conflict does occur at Cedar House, but such events are rare and quickly resolved, by the police if necessary. Most patients are in fact quite vulnerable and not the least bit aggressive. The doors at Cedar House are not locked, but patients are permitted to depart only with a pass. The open-door policy is successful in operation and in further contributing to the feeling of normalcy.

We observed that the quality of food is definitely inversely proportional to the size of the institution. Our son has often commented that the food at Cedar House is good. It is homemade and prepared in the Cedar House kitchen, which is open to the patients at all times. It is cooked just prior to meal time as it would be in any household, and the patients eat dinner together at two large tables in the kitchen—quite different from the hospital cafeteria style.

Case 2

A 41-year-old businesswoman was transferred into treatment at Cedar House from a psychiatric hospital where she had been under the care of a private psychiatrist for several months. Shortly before her hospital admission, she had entered outpatient treatment with the private psychiatrist. At that time she was planning to marry, give up her business, and move to a new city. She complained to the psychiatrist of emotional instability and binge eating. She reported somewhat unstable personal relationships: when she was younger she had lived in a commune and had led a life of hitchhiking and free sexual behavior. The psychiatrist began to treat her with fluoxetine hydrochloride (Prozac), but, within hours of the first dose, she reported agitation and racing thoughts. Her psychiatrist diagnosed bipolar illness (manic) and admitted her to the hospital.

In the hospital, the patient appeared to lose her self-control. She repeatedly banged her head against the wall, and, when she did this, she was placed in restraints. She was regarded as dangerous to herself because she threatened suicide, made superficial cuts on various parts of her body, and said that if she were released she would drive her car fast. She reported occasional strange visual hallucinations, such as seeing a zebra on a Colorado mountain trail. She failed to improve with treatment with medications and was eventually treated with seven different drugs; she became so oversedated that she had to receive them on a seven-times-a-day dosage schedule. Her health insurance benefits ran out after several months of treatment in the hospital, and she was referred to the mental health center with a recommendation that she receive ECT.

The mental health center admitted her to Cedar House, where her diagnosis was changed from bipolar disorder to personality disorder with histrionic features. At Cedar House, she was expected to demonstrate self-control and help with routine daily chores. She was given reassurances that she did not have a serious mental disorder and was gradually weaned off her medications. During the early days of her admission she would, at times, bang her head against her bedroom wall. The staff response was a low-key request that she not do this. She also kicked a hole in the wall and broke a window; she was billed for these damages.

Within a week the patient was showing less attention-seeking behavior and was beginning to discuss the various stresses in her life in psychotherapy. She was given passes to visit her home and work part-time, and, after 2½ weeks at Cedar House, she was discharged to outpatient care with the mental health center. She regained her former level of functioning, returned to work, and dropped her plan to marry and move. Five years later, she continues to do well and is not in psychiatric care.

This is the patient's description of her experience at Cedar House:

At first, for a variety of reasons, it was difficult for me at Cedar House. Having spent the past weeks in a hospital under suicide watch, often in solitary, I had become dependent on being contained. I had turned inward and given myself up as hopelessly psychotic; but that was fine with me: I wanted no part of the threatening world around me. Besides, I had been a prep-school-bred "captain of industry" with well-bred and monied friends: I was loath to live in a house full of fearful people to whom I had previously felt superior.

My feelings seemed well-founded when I walked in with my battalion of nurses from the hospital. The furnishings were clean and well-used, but what I saw was poverty. The people were busy with chores or reading, but I saw back-alley drug users, transients, murderers, and rapists. The staff, I told myself, were only there because they couldn't get "real jobs." This new doctor and therapist, moreover, were clearly out of touch with reality.

I soon realized I was going to be challenged. I was moving from a comfortable but ineffective traditional therapeutic approach into an arena of "tough love." I could not engage these people in the ghoulish world I wanted to create. Didn't they know that I was sick? What was wrong with them? My defenses and games became useless and counterproductive. I was held accountable—no bullshit allowed—but I understood that the "hard line" was accompanied by genuine support and caring. I was gently but firmly nudged along. I felt put upon by the reality of doing chores, but began to sense a change. Instead of directing my energies into being crazy, I was able to direct them into something productive. Empowerment was being used to heal.

I began to notice my housemates—from those with scant internal resources to the truly gifted. The community was important: it got me out of my head and into my life. The door of the house was open, and I could venture into the outside world to test myself. Can I take the bus? Do I want to run away? From sessions with my therapist, I was able to develop self-discipline and self-love. Living at Cedar House was like growing up in a healthy family—the care and no-nonsense focus on responsibility allowed me to emerge as an adult capable of taking care of myself again. I don't know if it was the caring, the therapy, the requirement to grow up, or the open door to the outside world that contributed most to my recovery. They were woven together into a fabric of real life that offered protection, direction, and momentum, which allowed me to walk out the door and back into my life.

Conclusion

Locked doors, seclusion, and restraints are unnecessary for the large majority of people who need acute psychiatric care, and their use may, in some cases, make matters worse. For suggestible patients like the one in the last case described, for patients with borderline personality disorder, and for many patients with psychosis, the confinement of the hospital unit can engender loss of control and increase the risk of aggressive or self-destructive behavior.

The normalizing atmosphere of a domestic alternative to the psychiatric hospital has a number of benefits—a less alienating environment for patients and staff alike, cues for the patient to function with as little pathology as possible, opportunities for reintegration into normal community activities and, it emerges, better food—all for a quarter of the cost of traditional hospital treatment. When health care reimbursement mechanisms catch up with the state of the art in community psychiatry, the domestic alternative to hospital care may well become a popular approach to acute psychiatric treatment.

Reference

Brook BD, Cortes M, March R, et al: Community families: an alternative to psychiatric hospital intensive care. Hosp Community Psychiatry 27:195–197, 1976

Venture: The Vancouver Experience

Editor's Note

VENTURE, AN ACUTE TREATMENT FACILITY IN VANCOUVER, BRITISH Columbia, is similar in several important ways to the program described in the previous chapter. Like Cedar House, it is an open-door household with an informal, relaxed atmosphere, yet offering close supervision. Residents are encouraged to do household chores and may leave to run errands and take care of business matters. The facility is under the same administration as the local community mental health teams and provides good continuity of care; psychiatrists and staff of the community programs come to Venture to provide treatment for the acutely ill patients.

Venture serves a large urban catchment area and, at 20 beds, is larger than Cedar House. The authors comment that the increase in cost-effectiveness that comes with the larger size is at the expense of certain environmental benefits associated with a more homelike, small-scale setting.

Chapter 2

Venture: The Vancouver Experience

Nicholas Sladen-Dew, M.B., Ch.B., M.P.H., F.R.C.P.C.
Anne-Marie Young, R.N.
Hugh Parfitt, M.B., F.R.C.P.C.
Rollande Hamilton, R.P.N.

*T*here are several advantages to providing acute psychiatric care in a residential facility firmly rooted in the community. First, a noninstitutional setting provides a more normalizing environment for those patients who do not need the structure and supervision of a hospital ward. Second, a residential setting is closely attuned to the social milieu in which the patient normally functions and will cause less disruption to the delicate links of community networks (Okin 1985; Polack 1978; Stein et al. 1975). Third, there is a significant cost advantage. Yet despite these benefits, there is a reluctance in North America to take full advantage of programs that offer a level of care midway between hospital treatment and community-based case management.

In this chapter, we examine some of these issues from a Canadian perspective, drawing on 17 years of experience with Venture, a short-term acute care psychiatric residence in the community.

We begin with a brief overview of Venture's parent organization, because what little success Venture has achieved is largely based on how it relates to the system as a whole, as well as its intrinsic characteristics. We then describe Venture's admission criteria and treatment program. Finally, we touch briefly on staffing and costs, and we conclude with a discussion of Venture's key ingredients.

We acknowledge the assistance of our Research Assistant, Lianne Fisher, and the contribution of Stephen Bornemann, M.S.W., M.P.A., Director of the Broadway South Mental Health Team, GVMHS.

Venture's Relationship
With the Mental Health System

The Greater Vancouver Mental Health Service (GVMHS) is a non-profit society that, for the past 20 years, has coordinated the provision of community mental health services to an urban population of approximately 700,000 (Sladen-Dew et al. 1993). GVMHS receives global funding from the Province of British Columbia and has considerable latitude in program development to respond to local community needs. This arrangement has provided GVMHS with the flexibility to develop what has recently been described as one of the more comprehensive and well-integrated urban community mental health services in North America (Torrey et al. 1993).

GVMHS accepts 7,000 new referrals each year and carries an active caseload of approximately 4,000 mentally ill adults, the majority of whom are chronically mentally ill (50% of the patients have schizophrenia). Each year about 700 patients are hospitalized and almost the same number of patients are admitted to Venture. GVMHS delivers its basic service through community mental health teams, each situated in one of nine geographic catchment areas. The teams provide case management (with physician support) at a patient-to-staff ratio of about 40:1. Information and referral services plus triage, quick response, and a variety of team-based rehabilitation and social programs are also provided by the teams.

Several support services at separate sites assist the teams in fulfilling their mandate, with Venture being one of these. Others include the Mental Health Emergency Service, which provides city-wide psychiatric assessment and treatment outside of normal working hours; the Mental Health Residential Service, which organizes a variety of housing programs; a Multicultural Liaison Service; and a Dual Diagnosis Program. GVMHS also coordinates the work of 13 nonprofit societies that provide additional drop-in, vocational, and housing programs throughout the city.

Venture was created in 1975 as a 10-bed facility to provide primarily short-term crisis resolution. One of the keys to Venture's effectiveness is its development in direct response to the needs of the patients and staff at the community mental health teams. The Venture program was initially located in a renovated house in the central part of Vancouver. Over the 18 years since its inception, the demand for this service and the level of acuity of the team patients' illnesses have increased. The teams have found that many of their patients can be satisfactorily treated in the Venture setting, rather than in the hospital. In 1990, Venture expanded to 20 beds and was moved into a facility built for its purpose.

Because Venture is under the administration of GVMHS, it shares with the community mental health teams a similar philosophy and approach toward patients. Many staff members at Venture have taken positions on the community mental health teams. Venture has developed positive links with staff at the teams: their patients and staff perceive Venture as providing practical assistance without distancing patients from their community treatment base.

Although the primary link is between Venture and the community mental health teams, an important secondary link exists between Venture and the Psychiatric Assessment Unit (PAU), situated adjacent to the emergency room of the Vancouver General Hospital. This PAU is the primary hospital-based psychiatric assessment unit in the city. It can admit patients on an involuntary basis for assessment and treatment. The average length of stay in the PAU is 5 days, after which patients are discharged to the community, transferred to a psychiatric inpatient unit, or discharged to Venture. Because of its strong connection with the teams, Venture accepts patients from the PAU only when they are eligible to be registered with GVMHS. Venture's willingness to assist the hospital in this way promotes a positive relationship with the hospital, so that when the need arises to transfer a patient from Venture to the hospital, it is usually accomplished without delay. This relationship also allows Venture to admit acutely ill individuals on a trial basis, knowing that it has the backup of the PAU.

Description

As previously mentioned, Venture's goal is to provide a level of care that is intermediate between community case management and hospitalization. This is achieved by creating an informal, homelike atmosphere with sufficient structure and intensive staffing to provide an opportunity for patients to resolve their acute psychiatric crises.

Venture is now a 20-bed house situated on a corner lot in a residential neighborhood. The ground floor has smoking and nonsmoking communal areas with a fireplace, paintings, comfortable sofas, and soft lighting. A kitchen, dining area, and outside patio with picnic tables and a barbecue are available for patients. Patients are given either single or shared rooms, depending on availability and preference. On a lower level are laundry facilities and an exercise and recreational area. Rooms are provided for staff charting and files and for private interviews, but staff spend most of their time with patients in the common areas.

Referral and Continuity of Care

Venture was created mainly to serve the patients of GVMHS. As a result, 70% of admissions to Venture are referred by the nine community mental health teams. The remainder are evenly referred by the Mental Health Emergency Service and the hospital settings (notably from the PAU).

When patients move from one treatment setting to another, continuity of care is frequently disrupted. At Venture such discontinuities have been reduced to a minimum. Venture staff assign overall clinical responsibility to the case manager and physician who normally look after the patient at the community mental health team. Continuity is also preserved because staff at Venture and at the mental health teams share a common, underlying community treatment philosophy.

In practice, the team admits a patient to Venture and a Venture staff member is assigned. Meetings take place with the patient, Venture staff, and the mental health team to plan treatment goals and strategies. People in the patient's support network in the community (e.g., boarding home operators and family members) are also invited to take part in this process. The patient can be discharged from Venture much earlier than if the patient had been admitted to a hospital because of this strong continuity of clinical care. A patient with residual psychotic symptoms may even be discharged to a supportive home setting. Obviously, this can only be done if staff have a thorough knowledge both of the patient's home situation and of the acute manifestations of the illness.

The concept of continuity of care, however, goes beyond providing consistent clinical responsibility across treatment settings. Continuity of care also implies the maintenance of valuable connections between the patient and the network of supports in the community. Programs like Venture, which are situated close to the neighborhood in which patients live, are able to preserve and, at times, to strengthen the fragile links between the patients and their support network.

Admission Criteria

Criteria for admission to Venture are flexible. They take into consideration the referred patient's characteristics, staff workload, and the mix of patients in the house. Often patients are admitted on a trial basis. Many patients, who might otherwise have been admitted to a hospital, have been effectively treated at Venture. Nevertheless, 20% of patients are eventually transferred to a hospital from Venture because their behavior continues to be so disturbed that it would be unsafe to manage such patients in an open-door facility.

The success in admitting patients on a trial basis, and to do so with safety, depends on relatively high levels of professional staffing and a close link with the hospital so that transfers can be expedited when they are necessary. Venture does not substitute for hospital care when a patient requires either greater structure or a comprehensive psychiatric and medical evaluation involving the full diagnostic resources of a hospital.

Patients are not excluded from access to Venture on the basis of diagnosis. However, there is a strong emphasis on serving those with a chronic mental illness. Twenty-eight percent of the patients have schizophrenia, and a further 46% have another psychotic disorder, such as bipolar or schizoaffective disorder, a brief reactive psychosis, or a psychotic depression. Seventeen percent are admitted with psychotic symptoms, such as delusions or hallucinations, as the primary complaint. The remainder are admitted with symptoms of anxiety and dysphoria, secondary to social stressors. Twenty percent are admitted with low to moderate levels of suicidal ideation. Fifteen percent of patients are admitted in crisis with a primary Axis II diagnosis of personality disorder. Venture does not admit patients with dementia or delirium.

Also excluded from admission are patients at high risk for suicide and those so disorganized that they require the close supervision of a hospital inpatient unit. Patients with a history of violence are not necessarily excluded, but those with a history of violence in the past 24 to 48 hours are carefully screened prior to admission. Patients who meet the dangerousness criteria of the Mental Health Act for involuntary admission are not admitted to Venture, but are sent directly to the hospital. Also excluded are patients who have a long history of heavy drug or alcohol abuse in the recent past and who are at high risk of chemical withdrawal. Patients with a serious psychotic illness who have abused alcohol on one or two occasions in their recent past are usually admitted. The incidence of alcohol and substance abuse is high among seriously mentally ill people, and to exclude patients from the benefits of Venture because of concurrent substance abuse is considered too restrictive.

Treatment

The objectives of the treatment program at Venture are the reduction of symptoms, the resolution of crisis, and the rapid reintegration of the patient into the community. The expectation is that the length of stay will be short and that the patient will be able to return to full or partial (transitional) functioning in the community. The mean length of stay at Venture is 8 days, with most patients spending 2 to 3 days, and a small number staying in excess of 2 weeks. The most important element of treatment is the structured but informal, low-stress milieu. It is a place where patients can experience a period of rest that allows them to distance themselves from stresses in the community. Patients and families have remarked that even a few days of respite are welcome, and that this intervention has seemed to reverse an incipient decompensation before hospitalization becomes necessary.

The Venture staff provide 24-hour assessment of symptoms and level of functioning. They carefully monitor medications, because poor medication compliance is often associated with relapse. They communicate their observations to the patient's case manager and physician at the mental health team, and they all work together to adjust the treatment plan.

In keeping with Venture's philosophy, an overly programmatic and institutional approach is de-emphasized. Venture staff do not become involved in intense psychotherapy sessions with patients, and they avoid confrontational group therapy. Similarly, a patient does not engage in formal rehabilitation programs at Venture. Venture, however, does provide recreational and social activities to which patients are invited but which they are not required to attend. When patients begin to show signs of stabilization, they are asked to take on daily chores at the house. Patients are also encouraged to go for walks in the community, to run errands, or to return to their homes to retrieve belongings or to tend to important business matters. This system encourages patients to maintain links with their natural support systems.

Occasionally patients have difficulty establishing self-control, and this poses a challenge for residential programs. Venture does not have a locked-door policy, and patients cannot be prevented from leaving if they wish to do so. As a first step, staff attempt to defuse the situation by offering the patient a quiet area where the staff can administer one-to-one support and, when indicated, medications. This approach has worked well for the majority of patients. However, if the behavior escalates to a point where the situation is considered to be unsafe, Venture will call for emergency backup either from the mental health team or the after-hours on-call physician. In some instances, the patient will be hospitalized.

The ability to manage emergencies depends on the experience of the professional staff, a close relationship with the mental health teams, and the ability to arrange the transfer of patients to the hospital quickly. Despite the high level of acuity of the patients' illnesses, Venture has had no attempted suicides and has had a very low incidence of other "unusual occurrences," such as an assaultive behavior.

Staffing and Cost

An important aspect of Venture's success is the quality of its staff. The most important qualification is a sound psychiatric background. Staff must be patient-centered and have a well-rounded knowledge of community resources; they should also be independent, energetic, and creative. The clinical staff at Venture comprises nurses and non-credentialed health care workers, in a three-to-one ratio. Nurses with psychiatric expertise are the backbone of the program. A psychiatrist provides services to Venture on 3 half-days per week, and on-call physician support is available evenings and weekends. Non-credentialed health care workers are individuals who have past work experience in settings such as boarding homes, emergency shelters, and crisis line centers, but who do not have formal psychiatric training. They bring to the treatment team a blend of warmth and good interpersonal skills that is welcomed by patients. Because of the autonomy and independence of the Venture environment, the staff are skilled at mental health assessment, crisis management, and working closely with community agencies. Venture is staffed 24 hours a day, over three shifts (7 A.M.–3:15 P.M., 3 P.M.–11:15 P.M., 11 P.M.–7:15 A.M.). Normally, four staff members work during the day and evening shifts, and three cover the night shift. Support staff include a manager and assistant manager, 1.5 full-time equivalent (FTE) secretaries, 1.5 FTE cooks, and 1.5 FTE housekeepers.

Although all staff members interact with the patients, each patient is assigned a primary staff member. The shifts are arranged to enhance continuity of care. Some observers have queried whether having up to 20 team therapists and physicians going to Venture to collaborate with staff might be overwhelming for both staff and patients. In practice, this has not been a problem. Venture staff do have meetings at shift changes, but there are no formal "ward rounds." Mental health staff and other professionals visit Venture throughout the day and evening.

With skyrocketing health costs, cost-containment measures are being sought. Many have argued successfully that programs such as Venture can provide high-quality treatment for many acutely ill patients who would otherwise have to be treated in a hospital. The per diem cost at Venture is $215CDN, compared with a hospital per diem of about $550CDN. Venture costs appear reasonable, even in light of employment of highly skilled staff, and the fact that the program is situated in a newly constructed building in a high-cost real estate city.

On a cautionary note, we have referred briefly to our decision in 1990 to expand from 10 beds to 20. A major factor in this decision was that it would be more cost-effective to run one larger facility rather than two smaller ones. There are some concerns that the qualities that made the smaller "old" Venture so successful, such as small scale and a more homelike environment, have not translated as well to the larger facility. Also, the size and layout of the new building sometimes have made it difficult for staff to keep track of the patients during the day. This has become a concern with the more severely disturbed patients. Most patients have commented that they enjoy the bright new facility, but some have said that they have found it "too busy," "too noisy," and "too crowded." In hindsight, we would have given serious consideration to building two 10-bed facilities and to adopting a slightly higher staffing ratio.

Discussion

Deinstitutionalization has increased the focus on providing effective care for individuals with chronic mental illness in the community. Nonetheless, this movement has not removed the perception that the hospital inpatient unit is the optimal environment for treatment of individuals who have acute exacerbation of psychiatric symptoms. Hoge and colleagues (1992) pointed out that terms such as "partial hospitalization" or "hospital alternative programs" are misleading because they focus attention on residential programs as a substitute for the hospital "rather than as a treatment in its own right or as the most appropriate intervention for certain patients or clinical conditions" (p. 346). In addition, Hoge and associates noted that the term "partial hospitalization" subsumes a vast array of programs and services. These include "day hospitals," "day treatment," and "day care" programs, many of which have failed to live up to their expectations (Rosie 1987). The rightful place for programs such as Venture has thus been obscured.

Similarly, there have been attempts to conceptualize Venture-type programs as "step-down" units of a hospital setting. This infers that patients must be admitted to an inpatient unit before they can benefit from a less intensive program. This highlights the point of Hoge et al. that community residential treatment facilities, not physically attached to a hospital, are not generally viewed as treatment programs in their own right.

We suggest that residential programs are best conceived as "step-up" units developed within the framework of community mental health services, responsive to those patients who are being looked after by standard or intensive case management. If hospital inpatient units were organized on a catchment area basis and were to incorporate a continuum of care model like Venture, then they might be better suited to provide short-term treatment for those patients who are either unable to be cared for in an open-door residential setting or who require tertiary care and treatment.

In the GVMHS system, 17.5% of the adult caseload is hospitalized each year (700 patients). This percentage has remained remarkably constant over the past few years, and we believe that it represents a figure that reflects a fairly well-integrated and comprehensive urban mental health system. Stein and Test (1980) argued that intensive case management can substitute for the role of partial hospitalization programs. Like many programs, GVMHS cannot afford the staffing costs associated with intensive case management for even a fraction of its 4,000 chronically mentally ill patients. We currently have over 600 admissions per year to Venture, and until further studies are undertaken, we can only speculate whether increasing the number of these programs would result in a reduction of the number of hospitalizations. It seems likely that some of the patients transferred to an inpatient unit after 5 days on the PAU might be as well or better served in a Venture setting. As Okin (1985) pointed out: "There is ample evidence that improvements in community programming can markedly reduce the rate of readmissions among discharged patients" (p. 744).

Using Venture to provide respite from social stresses and to provide extra support undoubtedly results in less need for hospitalization. This accords with Polak's 1978 proposition that "it is usually disturbances in small social systems around the patient that are the most frequent primary cause of admission, [and] it follows that direct intervention in the social environment of the patient should be the cornerstone of a comprehensive system" (p. 115).

Okin (1985) reiterated many of Polak's suggestions. Inevitably, patients need assistance in a community setting where they can develop the techniques necessary to maintain mental health adaptation (Okin 1985; Polak 1978; Stein and Test 1980).

Case Examples

Case 1

Ms. G. is a 32-year-old woman with a diagnosis of chronic schizophrenia and chronic polysubstance abuse. She is followed by her physician and case manager on one of the community mental health teams of the GVMHS.

Before her Venture admission, she had been briefly admitted to the hospital with an exacerbation of psychosis, probably connected with substance abuse. Following a brief admission, she was discharged to home, where she continued to abuse alcohol. This resulted in a further exacerbation of psychosis, culminating in an overdose of acetaminophen (Tylenol) and readmission to the hospital. Following a reduction in the level of her psychotic symptoms, Ms. G. was discharged to

Venture for a further period of stabilization. The treatment goals at Venture were aimed at providing a supervised setting, continued monitoring of mental status, and monitoring of both suicidal ideation and substance abuse.

On admission, Ms. G. described herself as "depressed and hopeless" and rated her mood as 2 on a 10-point scale. She reported that she felt that there were cockroaches in her body and stated that she could hear them talking. She denied suicidal ideation, and there was no evidence of substance abuse throughout her stay. Her mood gradually improved, and the delusions decreased. Ms. G. formed a good therapeutic relationship with the staff at Venture and was once again urged to seek drug and alcohol counseling, to which she halfheartedly agreed.

After a 13-day stay, Ms. G. was discharged, returning to her home and receiving homemaker assistance twice a week. She was also linked to various community drop-in services, and follow-up continued with staff at the community mental health teams. Her psychotic symptoms have been less intrusive and more tolerable, and her drug and alcohol use has not been a problem since she accepted substance abuse treatment.

Case 2

Mr. J. is a 34-year-old man living alone in Vancouver's downtown "skid row" area. He is followed by the community mental health team serving that area and has a diagnosis of schizophrenia.

Mr. J. was referred to Venture when the team learned from the hotel manager that Mr. J. was yelling and giggling to himself at night, hitting himself in the face, vomiting on the rugs, and plugging the toilets.

Following consultation with the team case manager and physician, Mr. J.'s neuroleptic drug was increased, and he was provided with bedtime clonazepam (Klonopin). Other treatment goals included providing a supervised setting, assessing mental status, ensuring medication compliance, monitoring for self-inflicted injury, and assessing general level of functioning and activities of daily living skills.

Mr. J. settled well into Venture's routine and responded to the supervision and guidance. He mostly kept to himself, peripherally interacting with other patients. Mr. J. consistently denied having hallucinations, although he was often noted to be laughing or mumbling to himself and appeared preoccupied. His conversation was vague, and he had difficulty processing information.

There were no further episodes of self-injury or vomiting, and appetite and sleep patterns were adequate, yet his general level of functioning in terms of nutritional and self-care needs was severely lacking.

Following an 11-day stay at Venture, arrangements were made to secure a boarding home placement for Mr. J., to which he happily agreed. Once accepted and placed at the boarding home, the mental health team staff continued with community follow-up.

Conclusion

In this chapter we described a 24-hour professionally staffed residential program that provides a level of care for patients with serious mental disorder midway between case management and hospital treatment. The key ingredients in its success are

- Excellent continuity of care with the community mental health teams
- Effective hospital liaison
- Treatment that is tailored for each individual
- An environment that establishes an informal and relaxed atmosphere combined with close supervision
- A team of specially trained professional and noncredentialed staff
- The ability to adapt and keep pace with new demands from the mental health system

In this regard, Venture meets many of the characteristics identified by Bachrach (1980) in her review of model programs.

In addition, GVMHS and Venture have not experienced the problems of funding, integration of services, and primary responsibility of patient care that have frequently been cited in the literature as impediments to establishing high-quality community mental health services (Cutler et al. 1992; Deiker 1986; Lehman 1989; Marshall 1992; Okin and Dolnick 1985; Yank et al. 1992).

Perhaps the most important lesson, however, is that Venture and the community mental health teams function together under the single administration of GVMHS. They are able to provide continuity of care for patients, to support the advantages of community treatment by reducing costs while providing a more normalizing experience for the patient, and to preserve as much as possible the links between the individual and the community. Venture demonstrates that acute psychiatric treatment in a residential setting fills an important gap in the continuum of mental health services and deserves to be more widely employed.

References

Bachrach LL: Overview: model programs for chronic mental patients. Am J Psychiatry 137:1023–1031, 1980

Cutler DL, Bigelow D, McFarland B: The cost of fragmented mental health financing: is it worth it? Community Ment Health J 28:121–133, 1992

Deiker T: How to ensure that the money follows the patient: a strategy for funding community services. Hosp Community Psychiatry 37:256–260, 1986

Hoge MA, Davidson L, Hill LW, et al: The promise of partial hospitalization: a re-assessment. Hosp Community Psychiatry 43:345–354, 1992

Lehman AF: Strategies for improving services for the chronic mentally ill. Hosp Community Psychiatry 40:916–920, 1989

Marshall PE: The mental health HMO: capitation funding for the chronically mentally ill. Why an HMO? Community Ment Health J 28:111–120, 1992

Okin RL: Expand the community care system: deinstitutionalization can work. Hosp Community Psychiatry 36:742–745, 1985

Okin RL, Dolnick J: Beyond state hospital unitization: the development of an integrated mental health management system. Hosp Community Psychiatry 36:1201–1205, 1985

Polak PR: A comprehensive system of alternatives to psychiatric hospitalization, in Alternatives to Mental Hospital Treatment. Edited by Stein LI, Test MA. New York, Plenum, 1978, pp 115–137

Rosie JS: Partial hospitalization: a review of recent literature. Hosp Community Psychiatry 38:1291–1299, 1987

Sladen-Dew N, Bigelow D, Buckley R, et al: The Greater Vancouver Mental Health Service Society: 20 years' experience in urban community mental health. Can J Psychiatry 38:308–314, 1993

Stein LI, Test MA: Alternative to mental hospital treatment, I: conceptual model, treatment program, and clinical evaluation. Arch Gen Psychiatry 37:392–397, 1980

Stein LI, Test MA, Marx AJ: Alternative to the hospital: a controlled study. Am J Psychiatry 132:517–522, 1975

Torrey EF, Bigelow DA, Sladen-Dew N: Quality and cost of services for
seriously mentally ill individuals in British Columbia and the United States.
Hosp Community Psychiatry 44:943–950, 1993
Yank GR, Hargrove DS, Davis KE: Toward the financial integration of public
mental health services. Community Ment Health J 28:97–109, 1992

Chapter 3

Crossing Place, Washington, D.C.

Editor's Note

CROSSING PLACE EMPHASIZES THE HUMAN ELEMENT IN ACUTE TREATMENT. Drawing on the experience of the Soteria Project, a novel community for the treatment of early schizophrenia (described in Chapter 7), the household uses a therapeutic community approach. Staff and patients are involved in decision making, attempts are made to determine the social factors triggering acute episodes of illness, and the treatment program incorporates many psychosocial elements. The program operates as an independent agency, and a wide range of seriously disturbed patients are referred from the public mental health system.

Crossing Place, Washington, D.C.

Pauline Bourgeois, M.S.W., Ph.D.

*R*esidential alternatives to psychiatric hospitals for people in acute psychiatric crisis are relatively uncommon. Policymakers and mental health professionals have not been enthusiastic about providing funding and resources for these demedicalized facilities, despite clear research evidence that the clinical outcomes of alternative facilities are as good as, if not better than, hospitalization (Kiesler 1982; Straw 1982). Alternative programs are also less expensive. For example, the per diem rate at Crossing Place in 1992 was $156; at the Washington, D.C., public hospital, $450; at a Washington, D.C., nonprofit hospital, $900; and at a Washington, D.C., for-profit hospital, $1,200.

For the past 15 years, Crossing Place (Figure 3–1), a pioneer and leader in this arena, has worked effectively with seriously disturbed individuals. Established in 1978 in Washington, D.C., by Woodley House, a nonprofit mental health agency, Crossing Place has had over 1,200 admissions since its inception. Only 10% have had to be hospitalized from Crossing Place. Our psychosocial approach "aims to maintain a balance between an understanding of people's intrapsychic lives, their interpersonal relations, and the intersystemic influences on their functioning and to weigh properly the influence of each to bring about desired change" (Turner 1987, p. 397). Effective psychosocial practice must include knowledge and skills of all aspects of a patient's life. This practice also examines the significance of patients' and staff members' ethnic identities, the environmental realities of their lives, the political climate of the times, and how these variables help or hinder patients in achieving their goals. Crossing Place provides patients with an opportunity to resolve their crises in a supportive milieu that provides intensive one-to-one and small-group intervention and practical problem-solving assistance. In many ways, it operates as a temporary family.

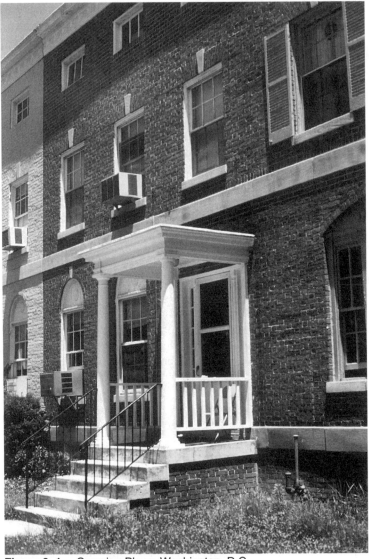

Figure 3–1. Crossing Place, Washington, D.C.

Background

Woodley House, a nonprofit agency established in 1958, has been a pioneer in establishing a 22-bed halfway house, a 51-bed supervised apartment program, a work training program with a thrift store, a self-help coffee house and referral program, and a model foster care program. Prior to the establishment of Crossing Place, when residents of the halfway house or apartment program required intensive psychiatric care, they were usually admitted to St. Elizabeths Hospital (the federal hospital that served as the District of Columbia's state hospital). This admission often meant loss of their apartments, entitlements, and ongoing activities, and disruption of their social networks. Because of these consequences, patients were unwilling to admit they were having serious difficulty or were in crisis. Program staff became discouraged because each hospitalization reversed the work done to help patients successfully integrate into the community. To solve this problem, Woodley House consulted Loren Mosher, M.D., who encouraged the staff to establish a community-based alternative to hospitalization, adapted from the successful Soteria model (Mosher and Menn 1978).

Political, economic, and judicial forces at that time converged to assist in the development of this alternative program. Washington, D.C., and the federal government were under court order *(Dixon v. Weinberger)* to provide patients at St. Elizabeths Hospital with a less restrictive alternative to hospitalization. The newly established Crossing Place quickly became a model alternative facility, thereby complying with the court order. Thus, Woodley House received public funding for Crossing Place to provide community-based crisis care in lieu of hospitalization.

Admission Criteria

Crossing Place's admission criteria include age 18 years and older, voluntary status, no serious complicating medical problem that requires hospital care, and a primary psychiatric problem other than substance abuse. Suicidal or assaultive patients are not excluded.

All patients are referred to Crossing Place by the Washington, D.C., Emergency Psychiatric Response Division (EPRD, gatekeeper to St. Elizabeths) or one of the Washington, D.C., community mental health centers. Other than bed availability, we are unable to ascertain what, if any, informal selection criteria are used by the heterogeneous group of referring psychiatrists. Private-pay patients are referred by their treating psychiatrists. In 1991, Crossing Place received a contract to serve hearing impaired patients.

Treatment and Operation

The Crossing Place brochure describes the therapeutic milieu and operation of this community-based program as follows:

- The basic therapeutic modality is one-to-one, intensive interpersonal support. Specially selected and trained staff members are with the patient for as long as intensive care and supervision are required. All staff members have experience in crisis care.
- The program's homelike environment is also an important therapeutic element: it minimizes the stress of entering residential care and returning to the community, because it resembles the patient's ordinary environment. Individuals focus on coping with their life crisis in a real-life setting. In addition, the small, intimate, and rapidly responsive environment, as well as the view that patients are responsible members of a temporary family, minimizes the potential for severe acting out.
- The staff members work closely with the director and psychiatrists to help individual patients formulate goals and plans. The entire staff meets regularly to discuss problems encountered in the helping process. The program director and psychiatrists are available to give individual attention to patients with particularly difficult situations.
- The length of stay varies from a few days to several months, depending on individual needs. Discharge is effected when the crisis has subsided and adequate plans have been worked out for important aspects of postdischarge living and treatment.

Originally, many professionals in the mental health community were skeptical of placing patients with acute crisis in a voluntary, open-door setting located on a busy Washington, D.C., street. During the first few years of Crossing Place's existence, staff had to market the program to convince the gatekeepers of St. Elizabeths Hospital and the staff members of the mental health centers that Crossing Place was, in fact, a safe and effective placement. Crossing Place's documented effectiveness (Bourgeois 1992; Kresky-Wolff et al. 1984) over the past

15 years and the Washington, D.C., mental health administration's commitment to provide treatment in the least restrictive environment have made believers out of an initially skeptical group of mental health professionals.

Presenting Problems and Population Served

In practice, Crossing Place accepts a heterogeneous group of mostly long-term public mental health system "veterans" with a variety of diagnoses.

Examples of presenting problems and reasons for referral to Crossing Place include

* Attempted suicide
* Severe depression
* Inappropriate and potentially dangerous behavior
* Command hallucinations
* Victim of violence or rape
* Major loss (e.g., divorce, death of relative)
* Problems with medication management
* Flashbacks of childhood sexual and physical abuse
* Threats toward government authorities
* Recent diagnosis of human immunodeficiency virus (HIV)
* Acute psychotic episode

An average 45.5% of all persons admitted to Crossing Place between 1981 and 1990 had serious substance abuse problems complicating their psychiatric crises (Bourgeois 1992). In the past 10 years, the number of patients with substance abuse problems, physical and sexual abuse, and homelessness and those without resources (i.e., income, housing, mental health treatment, and day activity) have increased dramatically. For example, only about one-third (36.4%) of all the people admitted between 1981 and 1990 had all four of the above-listed resources in place at admission (Bourgeois 1992). There has also been an increase in the number of "young-adult chronics"—people who have had little institutional experience. Finally, in the last quarter of 1992, one-third of the people admitted tested positive for HIV or had acquired immunodeficiency syndrome (AIDS).

Table 3–1 shows the data from two research studies: a 1982 study of the first 150 admissions (Kresky-Wolff et al. 1984) and a 1992 representative sample (25%), stratified by year, of all admissions to Crossing Place between 1981 and 1990 (Bourgeois 1992).

Statistics are necessary for funding and research purposes, but are not descriptive of the human beings they represent. We do not view our residents in diagnostic categories, but as unique individuals with life stories and problems that must be listened to, validated, and addressed.

Staffing

Crossing Place staffing is designed to maximize interaction and to minimize hierarchical relationships between staff and residents. "New staff members are selected by current staff, who look for characteristics such as emotional strength, ability to view patients positively, relationship skills (especially flexibility and tolerance), and perseverance" (Kresky-Wolff et al. 1984, p. 72). Staff have a sense of ownership because they make, in collaboration with the residents, all the day-to-day decisions regarding admission, treatment planning, and implementation. We attempt to ensure that the staff represent the ethnic

Table 3–1. Two studies of admissions to Crossing Place

	1982 study (%) (*n* = 150)	1992 study (%) (*n* = 220)
Diagnosis		
Schizophrenia	62	55.9
Affective disorders	26	34.5
Nonpsychotic	17	
Other		9.5
Gender		
Male	44	45.5
Female	56	54.5
Ethnicity		
African American	N/A	59.1
Other	N/A	40.9

Note. The age range for the 1992 study was as follows: 18–25 years, 18.6%; 26–35 years, 47.3%; 36–64 years, 30.9%; and 65+ years, 3.2%. For the 1982 study the age range was 14–74 years, with a mean of 32 years (SD = 12).

and gender characteristics of the residents so that patients will find someone with whom they can connect. Staff work in mixed gender teams and work two 24-hour shifts per week. This allows the staff to experience the complete rotation of a resident's daily activities. It also allows them to attend school or hold second jobs. Student interns from area graduate schools are included as members of the team.

Care and nurturing of staff are vital in this intensive program. Time is provided for staff to explore their feelings, ideas, and concerns to help ensure they are truly available to the patients. Staff participate in a weekly 3-hour consultation and training session during which they evaluate their work, seek guidance, and deal with staff issues. Recently, discussion centered around our work with a 20-year-old woman who had attempted suicide, was seriously depressed because of rejection by a boyfriend because she was HIV-positive, and had recurrent night-mares that she claimed were associated with her being present at the murder of a friend. Staff members' feelings of helplessness were addressed. We discussed our own prejudices and our own fear of dying. We then discussed ways to work with this woman. We invited a professional who works with AIDS patients to share with us what he knew about working with this population. We try to use all resources at our disposal to ensure that staff receive the support they need.

How Does It Work?

Patients are referred to Crossing Place by the Washington, D.C., mental health system or private psychiatrists. The staff on duty decide on admission and complete the initial intake, which includes the patient's statement of his or her goals and expectations of Crossing Place. The person is settled in the house. A Crossing Place consulting psychiatrist, with a staff member present, evaluates the patient within 24 hours of admission. This allows collaboration and exchange of ideas, observations, and information between staff and consultant. Consultants make recommendations, clarify medication questions, and use the opportunity for patient and staff education. At the evaluation, patients reiterate their goals and their expectations for their stay at Crossing Place.

Emphasis is placed on individual needs rather than on fitting the patient into the facility's program. Crossing Place was designed to meet the following criteria for effective settings for acute psychosis (Mosher and Burti 1989):

- Small (eight patients), homelike
- High staff-to-patient ratio
- High interaction, peer relationship orientation
- Real involvement of line staff and patients in decisions
- Emphasis on autonomy
- Value placed on preservation of personal power
- Focus on practical problems (e.g., living arrangements, money)
- Encouragement to use community resources
- Positive expectations
- Minimal hierarchy
- Encouragement to establish postdischarge contacts

The major focus of the staff in the first few days is to stabilize the patient and to obtain a complete biopsychosocial history. We believe there is a social precipitant for each crisis. Each person has a story to tell (some more believable than others). Understanding the underlying factors of each psychotic episode and exploring these with the person provide a mechanism for working through crisis situations. For example, a recent suicide attempt may have resulted from overwhelming guilt and shame because of past sexual abuse. Staff will encourage the person to talk about the abuse and teach the person a variety of techniques to deal with the fear, shame, and guilt. We take the time to understand the stressors and then assist in the search for alternative methods of dealing with the situations. Growth and healing can be achieved by a combination of belief in the power and goodness of the human spirit, by creating an atmosphere of mutual sharing, and by supporting each other. Weekly community meetings also allow residents to share and to work out any problems with living together.

Crossing Place becomes the hub for all treatment and case management. Meetings are set up with the resident's treatment team (psychiatrist, therapist, case manager) at the mental health center, staff at the day program, family, friends, and significant others. The resident is taught to take the lead role in all meetings, with Crossing Place staff playing a supportive role. If possible, regular family meetings take place at Crossing Place or in the family's residence if they are unable to come to the facility. Crossing Place not only works on resolving the crisis situation, but coordinates an effective support system that will allow the patient to return to community living. This includes, but is not limited to, ensuring that the patient has housing, income, mental health treatment, a day activity, and a social network. The staff uses advocacy, accompaniment, assistance in applying for entitlements, environmental manipulation, and systems management to accomplish this. Real-life accomplishments in these tasks help the patients and staff to develop problem-solving skills, assertiveness, self-esteem, and self-empowerment. Table 3–2 shows examples of staff techniques and interventions.

Relationship, earthiness, and optimism are the keys to working with this population. Emphasis is placed on patients' strengths and their ability to participate in their own treatment. Attempts are made, and are usually successful, to bring the patient's entire network system, including family, roommates, and significant others, to meet with the patient and staff as assistants to help resolve the crisis and arrange aftercare. Staff members coordinate all aspects of the patient's treatment and regularly communicate with the patient's psychiatrist, therapist, and case manager.

Case Examples

A look at two cases will give an idea of the complexity of patient problems and the use of sometimes unorthodox interventions employed by staff for stabilization and assistance in the attainment of patient goals.

Case 1

Ms. A is a 35-year-old West African woman referred to Crossing Place by the Multicultural Mental Health Center. She had to be forcefully removed from a shelter because of her bizarre and destructive behavior. In the process of eviction, she physically attacked a police officer. Her symptoms had been diagnosed at different times in the past as chronic paranoid schizophrenia, bipolar disorder, and schizoaffective disorder. She had a history of alcoholism and anorexia. When Ms. A arrived at Crossing Place, she was very psychotic, agitated, fearful, mistrustful, and overly polite. She stated that she wanted to "return to her native land." She was afraid that she would die on the streets of the United States, homeless. Although she agreed to take lithium as prescribed, she absolutely refused to take any neuroleptic medication. She also refused to allow staff to contact her two family members who were in Washington, D.C. A citizen of a West African country, she had given her passport to her embassy for updating, and it had not been returned. She wanted to obtain her passport, purchase a plane ticket, and return to the country that she had left at an early age. Ms. A gave us permission to secure her records from five hospitalizations and from an outpatient

Table 3–2.   Staff techniques and interventions

Supportive techniques
- Provide asylum, protection, containment
- Control stimulation when necessary
- "Being with" and "doing with"
- Networking
- Advocacy with treatment teams, agencies, families
- Accessibility—24-hour phone response
- Role modeling
- Case management—assessment, planning, linkage, brokering, monitoring, evaluation, data gathering, mediation

Education and skills training
- Daily living skills
- Community education
- Money management, budgeting
- Nutrition
- Assertiveness training
- Stress management
- Anger expression and management

Therapeutic techniques
- Crisis intervention
- Milieu therapy
- Group and individual therapy
- Family meetings
- Expressive—breathing, grounding, meditation, guided imagery, movement, psychodrama, role playing
- Audiovisual—art, films, videos
- Cognitive-behavior therapy
- Psychodynamic

Other
- Educating and training professionals in the United States and foreign countries
- Training social work students and psychiatric residents

clinic at which she had received services.

The staff was faced with a variety of issues that needed to be resolved: 1) Did she really want to return to her homeland or was this merely a psychotic presentation of her desire to live in a safe place? 2) If we supported her plan and she did not follow through, she might be homeless again. 3) Could we work effectively on concrete plans with her? 4) If she continued to refuse medication, was hospitalization an option?

We had to coordinate all aspects of her treatment and implement goals. We met with her treatment team (psychiatrist and case manager) at the mental health center, who had been working with her for several months, to get information and to coordinate tasks. We learned that, in conjunction with her family members in Washington, D.C., several years ago arrangements had been made for her to return to her country, but at departure time she refused to board the plane. Her family still wanted to be involved. However, she refused to have any contact with them. Her fear of homelessness and death had increased so dramatically after her stay in the shelter that the entire team agreed to support her plan if she accomplished the necessary tasks for the trip. She agreed. Her treating psychiatrist again recommended a trial of a neuroleptic drug, which she adamantly refused. She stated that, if not taking the medication meant she had to leave Crossing Place, she would leave. She would then work on her plans while living on the streets. Because she was not a danger to herself or others, she could not be hospitalized against her will. We agreed that she could stay at Crossing Place, and we would assist her in returning to her homeland.

A multifaceted strategy was put into effect, which included plans for her return as well as an alternative if she failed to follow through. We decided to set in place a plan for housing, thus allowing her the option at every step of the way to change her mind and still have a safe place to live if her plan did not work.

Supportive treatment.   During the entire stay, the psychosis was evidenced by her constant outbursts at her voices and her need for cleanliness. Staff taught her relaxation techniques and did breathing exercises with her. Her fear of being evicted after an outburst was assuaged when staff tolerated the outbursts, sought the underlying reasons and stressors, and then taught her ways to express, contain, or control them. As she became more comfortable, she was able to express her fears of living in the United States as well as her fears of returning home. Acknowledging that the fears were real and that the decision she was making was a very difficult one, but could be changed at any time, helped her to focus on the tasks needed to achieve her goals. All options and alternatives were examined. To satisfy us, she agreed to interview for mental health housing.

When she became suspicious of food preparation, she was invited to cook and/or help with meal preparation. On days that she could not tolerate eating with the group, she ate with a staff member or alone in the kitchen. Her compulsive need for cleanliness and washing was addressed, and limits were placed on her use of the washing machine. For her, control and independence were issues. She refused to put her money in our safe. We feared she might spend it and not have enough to purchase her ticket. We negotiated an arrangement whereby she gave us a weekly bank statement. This satisfied both our needs and provided her a modicum of trust and independence.

As the time for her departure approached, Ms. A became more agitated with loud outbursts about her fear of the military and about being taken prisoner when she returned home. A student intern read the history of her native country and learned that there was a military coup at approximately the same time she left the country as a child. She was a member of the ruling family and her family was deposed. We hypothesized that she was probably a witness to the coup. This enabled us to deal with her very real fears and to understand her plight.

Advocacy and accompaniment. Staff played a major role in working with the ambassador to facilitate her return. At our first meeting he told us he knew Ms. A and her family. He knew that her mother, whom she had not seen since childhood, wanted to help. Arrangements were made for her to telephone her mother long distance. She did and her mother assured her the family would meet her at the airport and care for her on her return.

Staff accompanied her to get necessary photos, immunization shots, the plane ticket, and clothes. Several trips were made to the embassy to complete the necessary paperwork. The ambassador offered to see her off at the airport.

We contacted the airline for information and assistance. A week before her scheduled departure, the staff accompanied her to the airport to familiarize her with the surroundings and the process. A staff member prepared an itinerary for her and a step-by-step guide of what to do on the airplane, how to practice relaxation exercises on the plane, and how to get help if needed.

Staff concerns. The final few days before her departure were difficult ones for her and the staff. She became increasingly agitated, wanted to move out and wait in a hotel, washed constantly, and put plastic bags over her feet and legs to avoid contamination. Throughout the process we struggled with our decision to support this endeavor. Were we on the right track? Were we being professionally ethical? We debated these issues the entire length of her stay. We wondered if she would make it. We questioned her options. If she remained here, she would probably end up in a shelter or on the streets. If she did not leave as planned, we would then, at least, have some leverage for suggesting mental health housing and a structured day program. We decided in favor of supporting her decision to leave.

The day before she left we met again and assured her that if she wanted to change her mind, if the pressure of the return was too great, we would help her with housing and treatment in the United States. Her reply was "I know you think I'm very psychotic and incapable of making a decision. However, you must understand my fear: that is what is making me so upset. I know that if I stay in the United States, I'll end up dead on the streets. I am afraid of returning home because I fear the military will capture me before I can be with my family. I know going back will be difficult, but my family is there and that is where my stepmother went when she was very sick, and that is where she died."

We made arrangements with the ambassador to meet her and a staff member at the airport so she would feel fully supported. All her medical records had been sent to her home country so her family could obtain the mental health treatment she needed. Although she was agitated and fearful, Ms. A greeted the ambassador at the airport, met with the airline personnel, and made the trip to her homeland. The next day the ambassador informed us that 20 members of her family greeted her upon arrival. He assured us she would be well cared for.

Case 2

Mr. B is a 55-year-old man who was referred to Crossing Place by the EPRD with a diagnosis of psychotic disorder. He had been brought to the EPRD by the staff of a homeless shelter because he had inadvertently overdosed on his medication and was considered a danger to himself. At the EPRD, he was interviewed by the referring psychiatrist, injected with a dose of haloperidol, and referred to Crossing Place. They gave us very little information about this man. "See what you can do and find out about him" was the request they made to Crossing Place. He was described as confused and anxious, with grandiose religious delusions, and he admitted to hearing voices.

In his initial meeting with Crossing Place staff, the information he provided appeared to be distorted and inaccurate. He stated that he had been brought to Washington, D.C., from another state by a man who was arrested for stealing checks. Since then, he had been living on the streets, and, occasionally, when things got bad, he stayed at a shelter. He also stated that he was born on a "peanut farm school" in the country (which turned out to be a dirt farm) and that his parents had died in 1850. He claimed that he was in the army, navy, marines, and air force during World Wars I and II, and the Vietnam War. He appeared to be a refugee with limited skills from the back wards of a state hospital. The possibility of organicity due to alcoholism was considered.

Crossing Place's consulting psychiatrist provided the staff with the following notes:

> Mr. B is bizarrely dressed, unkempt, and unable to track at all. He is an impossible historian. He hallucinates, is completely disoriented to time, date, and place; could not recall three objects; and denies suicidality. Recommendation: 1) piece together a story, 2) see if he is in the Veterans Affairs system, and 3) get some kind of records so we can figure out what's going on with him.

Mr. B presented as a frightened, disheveled individual whose manner of interacting was to preach the "good news" in a very loud tone of voice. His only belongings were scraps of paper he carried in a plastic bag. Because he lived on the streets and did not have an opportunity to bathe and shower, he looked more frightening than he actually was. After a shower, a change of clothes, and a badly needed haircut, he appeared more relaxed. He was very pleased with his appearance and was more receptive to the many questions staff had about his life history.

We had devised a system to handle his "preaching" because it could have become a major disturbance in our neighborhood. He was allowed to preach in the house until noon. Then the amount of time was reduced to an hour a day. Staff tried to divert his attention from preaching by assigning him tasks and just talking to him. Each day we tried to decrease the amount of preaching time. By the end of the first week, he had settled in and appeared to have more important things to do than preach—for example, talk with staff, figure out where he'd been, go for walks and outings, ride in the van (one of his favorite activities), and get a soda whenever possible.

The answers he gave during the first few days were confusing at best, and we wondered if we would ever piece anything together. The only clues we had were his scraps of paper and the information he provided. Each scrap of paper was examined for possible clues. He had a card from a state hospital from which we eventually received his records. He had cards with two different social security numbers. After two trips to the social security office, we discovered that he received social security and CHAMPUS benefits. We realized that he could also receive Supplemental Security Income (SSI), and he applied for it. He also applied for Medicaid. Within 3 weeks he received his back checks and had enough money for housing. He told everyone he was rich!

He was medicated when he arrived. At his intake at the community mental health center, he was given additional medicine (haloperidol). He became very tired, lethargic, and, sometimes, agitated and restless. Staff advocated with his psychiatrist for a reduction in medication. We believed that the environment would calm his agitation and make him more comfortable, thus reducing the need for medication.

Staff took him shopping and he bought clothes and personal items. He was happy. His delusions subsided and he became an integral part of the house. He learned and practiced daily living skills. We talked with him about a day program, and once he received Medicaid, he started a day program. He was very excited and proud that he was going to school and work each day.

During his time with us we found out that he could not read or write. He had headaches and we discovered he needed glasses. When he got his glasses he was sure he would be able to read! Staff coordinated his physical and psychological examinations and accompanied him because he was fearful of being reinstitutionalized. At one of the men's rap groups, he talked about being raped and beaten in the institution. He was happy with his new home and new-found friends.

Other residents in the house took charge of helping Mr. B settle in and learn to care for himself. He learned to interact with and let people know when his feelings were hurt. He became a willing participant in household activities and chores. When asked what he wanted at Crossing Place, he answered "love." This was a home where he was comfortable, accepted, and treated with respect.

Advocacy and system intervention.   Working with Mr. B presented many systems' challenges for staff. He was not exactly welcomed in the mental health system or in the mental retardation system. However, staff determination and skill at advocacy enabled this man to get the services he needed. Usually, the entire treatment network works together for the good of the patient. Although this case is an exception to the rule, it is important because it demonstrates that knowledge of laws, systems, and methods of advocacy are necessary.

The following are examples of several obstacles we encountered while attempting to obtain needed services.

- When we brought Mr. B to the mental health center for intake we found out that he had been there once before, but because they could not get any information from him, they did nothing. He returned to the streets with an appointment card. This time we interpreted and advocated for him. We helped set the wheels in motion for things such as treatment, housing, income, medical care, and glasses.
- At our second meeting, we informed the staff at the mental health center that we believed Mr. B belonged in the mental retardation system. We had made an appointment, but needed a psychological examination from the mental health center. It took almost 4 weeks of persuasion, followed by calls to the mental health center director, to receive the examination and the results.
- The mental retardation system evaluated him and told him it would be 6 months to a year before they could provide services.
- Mr. B exhibited signs of being overmedicated. He had received haloperidol intramuscularly. We advocated for a reduction in the amount of haloperidol and asked that he be given oral medication that we would monitor. It took several calls from Crossing Place staff and a call from our consulting psychiatrist to the prescribing psychiatrist to achieve our desired results. Once he received a lower dosage, he functioned better and was more willing to participate in daytime activities.

- The case manager was unwilling to find housing in the mental health system and advised us to return him to the shelter. We challenged this decision and warned that we would take the matter to the mental health commissioner and the newspaper, if necessary. Our advocacy caused intervention by the mental health administration, which told the case manager that sending this man to the streets or a shelter was not acceptable.
- Without our involvement the treatment team decided to return Mr. B against his will to the state where he had been institutionalized. We informed them that this was illegal and that we would intervene to ensure this did not happen. We asked the Dixon Monitoring Committee (the court-appointed group that oversees Washington, D.C.'s implementation of the Dixon Decree, which stated that patients had a right to live in the least restrictive environment) to convince the director of the mental health center of the illegality of sending Mr. B to another state against his will. This was accomplished. Mr. B had enough money to secure supported housing in a community residential facility. We found a home willing to care for Mr. B. The case manager was compelled to do the paperwork for this housing.

Mr. B found a home where he has been living very successfully for the past year. He attends a day program where he is learning carpentry. He calls us regularly and visits for meals and socializing. Without tremendous input from staff in advocacy and treatment, Mr. B would still be among the Washington, D.C., homeless population.

Summary and Conclusion

The operation of Crossing Place, a 15-year-old alternative to psychiatric hospitalization for people in severe psychiatric crisis, has been described. This eight-bed facility has admitted more than 1,200 long-term, seriously mentally ill, multiproblem "veterans" of the Washington, D.C., mental health system. Ninety percent are successfully returned to the community. There has never been a suicide. Its effectiveness is inexpensive when compared with psychiatric hospitalization: $156 a day versus $900 a day in Medicaid-eligible hospitals in Washington, D.C. To facilitate the process of recovery from crisis, the program stresses the importance of relationships with peers, staff, community-based team members, family, and friends. Its staff function in a variety of individualized roles with patients: "being with" to provide support and containment; "doing with" to access concrete resources; facilitation and advocacy with the treatment system and social networks; education in the areas of life skills, problem solving, and stress management; and therapy, utilizing a variety of verbal and expressive techniques.

The setting itself, an ordinary eight-room row house on a busy Washington, D.C., thoroughfare, lends itself to the creation of a family-like atmosphere that enables the program staff to use relationships to flexibly normalize, contextualize, and empower the experiences of patients in this unique setting.

References

Bourgeois P: The relationship between the continuum of changes in the context of metal health services, changes in clients admitted and service characteristics of an alternative to psychiatric hospitalization. Unpublished doctoral dissertation, Ann Arbor, MI, Northwestern University, 1992

Dixon v Weinberger, 405 F Supp 974 (D.D.C. 1975)

Kiesler CA: Mental hospitals and alternative care: noninstitutionalization as potential public policy for mental patients. Am Psychol 37:349–360, 1982

Kresky-Wolff M, Matthews S, Kalibat F, et al: Crossing Place: a residential model for crisis intervention. Hosp Community Psychiatry 35:72–74, 1984

Mosher LR, Burti L: Community Mental Health: Principles and Practice. New York, WW Norton, 1989

Mosher LR, Menn AZ: Community residential treatment for schizophrenia: two-year follow-up. Hosp Community Psychiatry 29:715–723, 1978

Straw RB: Meta-analysis of deinstitutionalization. Unpublished doctoral dissertation, Ann Arbor, MI, Northwestern University, 1982

Turner F: Psychosocial approach, in Encyclopedia of Social Work, 8th Edition, Vol 2. Edited by Minahan A, Becerra RM, Briar S, et al. Silver Spring, MD, National Association of Social Workers, 1987, pp 397–405

Chapter 4

Progress Foundation, San Francisco

Editor's Note

Progress Foundation in San Francisco, California, has established a series of acute treatment facilities that share many of the features of programs described in the earlier chapters. Steve Fields, who helped design and develop the Progress Foundation programs, describes the underlying principles that make households of this type distinctive and effective. They are small, normalizing establishments. Staff are selected as much for their life experience and their talent in working with others as for their specific professional training. Residents are involved in decision making, and the facility adapts itself to meet the needs of the patient. The author makes it clear that these are not mini-hospitals: in some ways these programs are the antithesis of standard treatment institutions, and they achieve results that hospitals cannot. There are inherent risks in running a human-scale program that does not respond to problems with a predetermined protocol, and this risk taking, the author argues, is a key issue in making treatment effective.

Progress Foundation, San Francisco

Steven L. Fields, M.P.A.

*I*n 1976, Progress Foundation, a nonprofit agency located in San Francisco, California, proposed the development of a short-term acute residential alternative to psychiatric hospitalization. At that time, there were few models on which to base this innovative service. The Soteria Project in nearby Santa Clara County offered some guidance, but that program was highly selective and focused on young, unmarried, newly diagnosed schizophrenic patients (see Chapter 7). The program designed by Progress Foundation was intended to serve all patients of the public mental health system, regardless of their length of time in the system, their diagnosis, or their prognosis.

The program that was developed and opened in 1977 was named La Posada. Implemented in conjunction with a transitional residential treatment program and a series of cooperative apartments, La Posada was the first nonhospital acute treatment program provided in a normalized, community setting for public mental health patients in California.

La Posada was designed to provide a community-based, social model equivalent to the inpatient unit for voluntary psychiatric patients. The goal of the program was to divert from the public system individuals presenting to psychiatric emergency rooms who would otherwise have been hospitalized as a result of an acute psychiatric episode. The program provided crisis stabilization, diagnosis and assessment, and treatment and rehabilitation based on a community support system model.

Since 1977, Progress Foundation has replicated the La Posada program three times. One program, Progress Place, is in Napa County, 45 miles north of San Francisco, and the home of the major northern California state hospital. The other two acute alternatives, Cortland House and Shrader House, are in San Francisco.

In addition to the acute residential treatment programs, the agency provides a full range of residential treatment services, including transitional residential programs that offer up to 4 months of structured treatment services, cooperative apartment programs, and permanent housing with support services. The agency mission is to provide a range of services that can prevent or minimize institutional care for persons with severe mental illness.

Background

The Progress Foundation acute residential treatment programs evolved directly from our "halfway house" services. The agency had provided transitional residential treatment services in three residences prior to the opening of La Posada. We learned that actively psychotic and suicidal individuals can be treated in a properly designed and staffed residential setting.

The goal of the three acute houses is to provide an equivalent to the hospital for individuals who require intensive support during a psychiatric crisis. La Posada, Cortland, and Shrader Houses in San Francisco and Progress Place in Napa County share a common treatment approach and program design, while maintaining unique characteristics that distinguish one program from the other. La Posada, for instance, has a bicultural, bilingual focus on Spanish-speaking patients. Cortland House has developed a program specifically for patients from the Asian community. Each of the houses reflects this cultural focus in specific staffing and program services, while also focusing on the overall goals of diverting individuals from inpatient hospitalization, or shortening the length of stay of those who require brief hospitalization.

The maximum length of stay in the acute houses is 2 weeks. Some individuals stay longer due to special problems with discharge planning and follow-up services. The average length of stay in the houses ranges between 9 and 13 days. Each program admits approximately 210 patients each year. The Progress Foundation acute programs strive to maintain a length of stay that is less than or equal to the local inpatient unit in order to accommodate new patients referred by emergency rooms.

Admission Characteristics

The programs serve slightly more men than women. This figure is influenced by the fact that the houses try to maintain some balance in the male-to-female ratio. If the programs did not provide control in this area, the houses would shift toward a predominantly male population. A majority of the patients in the San Francisco programs are from minority communities (52%), and approximately 19% identify themselves as gay men or lesbians. Close to 60% of the patients have severe substance abuse problems, and a growing number of referrals are positive for human immunodeficiency virus (HIV) or have acquired immunodeficiency syndrome (AIDS). This latter patient population, with acute and persistent psychiatric symptoms, substance abuse problems, and HIV- or AIDS-related complications, represents an emerging "triple diagnosis," which is having a major impact on the acute services. The problem is particularly intense when the acute programs attempt to find transitional residential treatment programs prepared to work with patients presenting with these complex issues.

The most recent patients in the acute houses reported an average of three hospitalizations within the 12 months prior to admission. The majority of patients have been hospitalized multiple times, and a growing number of patients report recent incarceration in jail, or they are referred directly from the jails to acute diversion.

To achieve the goal of minimizing the use of psychiatric hospital beds, all referrals to the acute houses come from the psychiatric emergency services, which also control access to inpatient beds. For diversion programs to have a direct impact on hospital utilization, admission to acute house beds must be controlled at the same triage point at which admission to the hospital beds is controlled. The acute residential treatment programs operate under a "no refusal" agreement with the referring emergency rooms. On rare occasions, an acute house may not be able to admit a particular patient because of specific situations in the program. For instance, a house may already have two or three patients on a "close watch" and cannot absorb another referral requiring one-to-one supervision. However, such instances are infrequent, and the programs strive to respond to any referral from the emergency rooms or inpatient units within 2 hours.

Treatment Programs

All of the acute programs provide a full, 24-hour program. Whereas some patients in the latter stages of their stay are beginning connections with day treatment services in the community, the majority of patients remain in the house and participate in an individualized day program designed to accomplish each person's treatment goals. The day and evening schedule is highly structured, with a combination of group meetings and individual counseling sessions, to develop, implement, and assess the ongoing treatment and rehabilitation plan. Each patient, to the level consistent with his or her ability, takes part in the functioning of the household.

Discharge planning begins as soon as the patient enters the program. In the initial, crisis stabilization phase, the counseling staff work with patients to focus on specific problems and potential plans and solutions. In the immediate, postacute phase of the crisis, patients begin to explore housing and treatment options in the community. As each patient approaches discharge, formal linkages are established with transitional residential settings, other housing options, and treatment resources in the community mental health system, such as vocational services, case management, individual therapy, and day treatment.

Staffing

To achieve the program goals, the staffing of the acute houses allows for a minimum of two counselors on duty for each shift. La Posada and Shrader House serve 10 patients, Cortland House has a capacity of 8, and Progress Place serves 7. During the most intensive treatment hours—8 A.M. to 10 P.M.—there are frequently as many as three or four staff members working with patients. Each acute house has a program director, a senior counselor, a day program coordinator, and 10 or 11 counselors. Each of the houses has a psychiatric consultant to advise staff and to provide training, consultation, and medication services for patients. The consultant is present approximately 15 hours each week. The psychiatrist is the only staff member required to have a specific professional mental health degree.

Treatment Philosophy

Beyond describing the specifics of the Progress Foundation acute programs, it is important to understand the programmatic and systemic philosophy that forms the basis for the services. It is easy to outline the details of a particular program—its staffing patterns, policies on medications, training program, or daily schedule of activities—and miss the essence of the program, its ethical underpinnings, and treatment philosophy.

In fact, practitioners in the mental health field are frequently too enamored with "model programs." We visit programs, soak up the atmosphere, gather up the forms, and rush back to our communities to re-create services that have had success in other areas. All too often, we find that our experience with the new program is disappointing, our results are less spectacular, and our enthusiasm wanes until we read or hear about a new, creative program.

This book contains the descriptions of several successful programs, each of which provides a residential, noninstitutional alternative to psychiatric hospitalization. The programs vary tremendously in their specific characteristics. Some are in urban settings, and others are in rural areas. Some have no medical personnel on staff at all, whereas others have a substantial component of medical care. Some are more institutional in their environment than others, with more rules and "traditional" staffing patterns.

The simple conclusion from this review of sample programs is that there is no single "model" for an acute residential alternative to psychiatric hospitalization. What has been successful in one community may not be possible or appropriate in another. Therefore, it is not always useful to describe a specific program in San Francisco, for instance, and assume that it is replicable in other communities, which face different challenges and realities.

It is helpful, however, to describe the philosophy and principles of a successful program. These elements can be translated into widely varying communities. Philosophy and principles travel across cultures and economic lines. The Progress Foundation programs have been successful because the services have followed a set of programmatic principles and have responded successfully to indigenous systemic issues and problems. The structures of La Posada and the other acute programs have evolved from these principles, and clinical practice is informed by these principles.

Acute Alternative Programmatic Principles

The following list of essential elements of the Progress Foundation acute residential treatment programs was derived, in retrospect, from the experience of developing La Posada. The initial development of that first acute program was driven by the challenge to serve acutely ill patients, a growing level of experience with increasingly difficult clinical problems in existing transitional residential programs, and an intuitive sense of what would work and what would not work in acute situations. Progress Foundation did not have a blueprint to follow.

After the initial program was a success, the agency leadership reviewed the process of trial and error and derived this set of guiding principles that formed the basis for all future program development within the agency. No single element of this list of principles is the unique discovery of Progress Foundation. Each of these elements has been discussed in the literature of community mental health and noninstitutional services. The combination of these familiar values represents the core of the acute alternatives to hospitalization at Progress Foundation.

Can the Progress Foundation acute programs serve everyone? The answer is no. But we have learned, over the years, that there is no single category of behavior that we cannot successfully treat. We have not been able to reach some individuals who, consequently, have required inpatient care, but patients who were violent at the time of admission, who were high suicide risks, who had recently set fires, and who were in the midst of an acute episode requiring constant supervision and support have been successfully admitted, stabilized, treated, and discharged.

Normalizing environment.   The single most critical aspect of the Progress Foundation acute programs is their homelike, human-scale environment. The residential setting provides an ideal framework for practical diagnostic work, skill assessment, and interpersonal interaction.

In the general mental health culture in the United States, we take our most frightened, most alienated, and most confused patients and place them in environments that increase fear, alienation, and confusion. Few would argue that hospital psychiatric wards represent familiar and reassuring environments for most individuals in psychiatric crisis. In fact, in most psychiatric institutions, staff and patients spend most of their day and their limited energy trying to overcome environmental barriers to make a human connection. In a field predicated on the establishment of relationships, we practice our trade in settings that are toxic to relationships and human interaction.

The premise of the Progress Foundation programs is that the homelike setting counters the patient's internal dissonance and confusion. The houses are designed to minimize the sense of environmental alienation; they are small (the largest Progress Foundation acute program serves 10 people), and the internal and external characteristics of the programs are similar to those of a household. A visitor walking down the street where a Progress Foundation acute program exists would find it difficult to discern which house is a mental health residential treatment setting.

In addition to providing this sense of belonging and familiarity, the residential environment offers a variety of opportunities to assess functioning, interpersonal behavior, and daily living skills. If the goal of an acute intervention is not just to stabilize, but to move an individual toward community living as soon as possible, the residential environment allows this reintegration to occur more naturally. From the beginning, patients are involved in the operation of the household and the manipulation of the environment as a part of their stabilization and treatment.

In the acute programs, patient participation in the operation of the household is an integral part of crisis intervention. We believe that the act of functioning, of focusing on a task such as preparing a meal or developing a shopping list, hastens stabilization and promotes healing during an acute crisis. Patients learn that they can experience disorienting thoughts and still function in their environment. Residential treatment settings offer this unique opportunity to utilize familiar, everyday tasks and challenges as tools in crisis stabilization and the restoration of functioning following an acute episode.

Patients are involved, from the point of admission, in the operation of the household. Teams of patients prepare the meals, along with staff. Patients and staff participate in the maintenance of the environment. Patient participation in this environment is real and relevant. Staff work and live among the patients. Offices are integrated into the general households, and staff spend most of their time in the midst of the house, interacting with patients.

The true "soul" of a residential treatment program can be found in the ritual of preparing, sharing, and cleaning up after a meal. In fact, dinner is probably the core "treatment" event in the acute houses because it involves the entire household in a common event. This activity can reveal more useful information about the level of functioning and capability of patients than most of the traditional groups and individual interviews that are also a part of the programs.

When Progress Foundation was designing the La Posada program, the mental health leadership in San Francisco, which was providing funding for the innovative program, was clear about its preference for an institutional setting. In fact, city officials had located an abandoned skilled nursing facility in the community that they believed would be ideal. Progress Foundation resisted these efforts, not because of our organizational opposition to institutional settings, but for a more practical reason: an acute alternative to hospitalization would not work as well in an institutional setting as it would in a normalized environment. The decision was based on our clinical judgment that we would lose too many assets by compromising the environment. We have not regretted our decision.

Multidisciplinary staffing.   Residential treatment programs unintentionally pioneered the idea of nonprofessional staff roles because the small, underfunded "halfway houses" of the early 1970s could not afford to pay professional mental health staff. As a result, agencies like Progress Foundation discovered the rich resource of men and women who did not have formal mental health training, but who brought to the program a wide array of skills, perspectives, and attitudes that enhanced the services.

In fact, when we opened La Posada, of the 12 original staff members, only 3 were experienced mental health professionals. One of the people with traditional experience was the half-time psychiatrist who helped conceptualize the program and who provided invaluable consultation to the staff. The staff included community activists who saw the program as an opportunity to provide service to the Latino community. Two counselors were poets who often performed their work in community coffee houses and churches. What we lacked in formal mental health training, we made up for in commitment, a willingness to learn, and a strong sense of purpose. Although a majority of the staff did not have formal mental health training, they had worked for Progress Foundation in other residential programs, and they brought that specific and valuable experience and perspective to the new program.

When Progress Foundation first proposed La Posada, city officials strongly encouraged the agency to utilize professionally trained staff. The funding levels for the program would have permitted such staffing.

Again, the agency had to examine, from a practical perspective, what staffing approach would work best. We concluded that a highly hetero-geneous staffing model, with traditionally trained professionals and nonprofessionals, was essential to the success of this program.

We have learned at Progress Foundation that *anyone* can be an excellent acute care worker, but not *everyone* can do the job. What this means is that our best staff have come from all walks of community life, and there is no single predictor of a quality acute care staff member. Above all, we look for individuals who are comfortable around patients in an open environment, and who are not afraid of the people we treat. If we had decided to eliminate the nonprofessional element of our staff, we would have lost many of our best staff members.

Working in an open, residential setting with acute patients places many demands on the staff. Many traditionally trained individuals are not comfortable with such an open environment. Progress Foundation has found that it is necessary to provide clear, specific training in the methods and practices of acute residential treatment for all of our staff. For many trained professionals, this represents a profound "retraining" effort. For those without such formal training, it is an opportunity to frame a new kind of community mental health experience.

Today, Progress Foundation's acute program staff are remarkably varied. Each staff consists of individuals who bring the essential ele-ment of professional training, as well as those who bring other kinds of life experiences. Over one-half of our acute program staff are from ethnic minority cultures. The staff speak more than 12 languages and dialects. We have priests, social workers, high school drop-outs, psy-chiatrists, poets, and a former circus performer among our valuable staff members. Ex-consumers of mental health services have regularly been a part of our staff, not in special roles, but in regular staff positions. In a synergistic way, the programs benefit from this broad range of perspectives and attitudes.

Another important element of this staffing model is that it is not hierarchical along lines of discipline. The staff works as a team. The program director is in charge of the service. The program psychiatrist carries no more weight in the program than a counselor. Program directors and counselors range from individuals with higher degrees in psychology or social work to individuals with no formal education since high school. This approach requires individuals who are comfort-able with such an egalitarian structure, who can find satisfaction in the results of the program rather than in a specific role or position of authority that is based on a degree or specialized training.

Patient involvement in decision making.   A central tenet of the Progress Foundation programs is that the patient is the expert on himself or herself. Staff, just because they have some clinical background and trained insight, should not make the mistake of believing that they know more about the patients than those individuals know about themselves.

In acute and crisis settings, when staff dictate treatment plans to patients, a lot of time is wasted. Many patients do not have the energy, the will, or the bad manners to argue with staff who "know what is best for the patient." As a result, patients often agree to treatment plans and goals that are not relevant to them, or that contradict their own sense of what they want or need. Often, in an acute crisis, patients have no legitimate idea what they want or need, and anxious, well-meaning staff substitute or create goals on behalf of patients. The end product of this process is that patients frequently fail to carry out treatment plans or neglect tasks that they have been assigned. Frustrated staff frequently blame the patient for this failure and label the patient "treatment resistant."

Successful acute alternatives approach the development of treatment plans differently. The patient is the primary source of information for developing any plans or goals. Even though the process may be frustrating or slow, the staff must remain focused on the stated intent of the patient. The role of the counselor in these situations is to suggest, guide, question, and challenge, but not to dictate or ignore.

When this principle is explained during staff training, I am frequently confronted with skeptical questions, such as: "What if the patient wants to be a brain surgeon? Should I just go along with that?" My answer is yes. After all, patients in an acute episode in our programs most frequently have no income, have no place to live or even sleep, are wearing the only clothes they own, and have not had any sustained periods of functioning for years. I would suggest that the steps that must be taken to assist the patient in becoming a brain surgeon are the same ones that would be taken under any circumstances. We need to work together to get a stable income, to find a decent affordable place to live, and to develop an array of support services in the community. It makes no difference whether their goal of being a surgeon is realistic, in the short run. Yet we argue about these kinds of issues all the time. It is the wrong argument, and it wastes precious time for the program and the patient.

The fundamental principle here is that patients will work to accomplish goals that they have had a central role in defining. The very process of listening to patients and taking their participation seriously is itself a way of promoting self-determination and focusing the intense effort of crisis resolution and stabilization on real problems and practical solutions.

Program flexibility and individualized treatment. Institutions are not flexible. It does not matter whether the setting is a 120-bed skilled nursing facility or a 6-bed group home; if the rules and structures are rigid, unchanging, and not subject to challenge, then the environment is an institution. Conversely, if any one patient or worker has the opportunity to change procedures, question authority, suggest new methods or ideas, and alter the culture of the program, then that environment is well on its way to being a true alternative to institutional care.

It is critical that acute residential treatment programs remain protean enough to break down their structures as often as necessary and to rebuild around the specific needs of the patient population, at any given time. Certainly, some procedures and rules endure because they have been proven effective and necessary after numerous challenges and reviews. However, programs must avoid the trap of continuing to do things because "that is the way we have always done it."

Progress Foundation programs make it a point of policy to review all rules, regulations, and program procedures on a regular basis, with the patients' involvement, to reaffirm their relevance or to discard those that are no longer necessary.

This programmatic flexibility extends to the implementation of individual treatment plans within the programs. By remaining small, the Progress Foundation acute programs can tailor the program response and treatment plan to each patient. Each patient presents with a unique set of circumstances on entering the acute program. With adequate numbers of staff, and with a programmatic ethic to treat each patient individually, the agency acute alternatives can develop specific plans, with varying discharge dates, and with a variety of treatment "packages" for each patient.

On any given day, the 10 patients in one of the acute houses could be engaged in as many as 10 different activities. New patients would be getting to know the household and stabilizing from the immediate acute episode. Patients in the middle of their 2-week stay might be involved in an aspect of the in-house program for a portion of the day and might be attending to business outside of the house at other times to establish housing, income, and other supports. Patients who are preparing to leave may spend much of their day linking with community programs that will provide their ongoing rehabilitation services. In the evenings, the programs offer a variety of groups that range from men's and women's groups to sessions that focus on the effects of medications or advocacy strategies with the Department of Social Services. Most groups are practical and focus on specific tasks or problems with developing community support services, such as housing, income, friendships, or vocational opportunities.

The commitment to flexibility must also extend to the overall treatment system. The Progress Foundation acute alternatives have a specific obligation to the treatment system of which they are a part to divert as many individuals as possible from inpatient treatment. Each program must continuously expand the range of patients it will treat. As patient populations shift, acute alternatives must also shift to remain effective.

One measure of the success of an acute alternative is if the next "wave" of patient problems shows up in the residential treatment program first. Shortly after opening, La Posada began to see the first signs of significant substance abuse problems in the patients referred from the emergency room at San Francisco General Hospital. By the time Cortland House opened 3 years later, dually diagnosed patients were permeating the system, and the acute houses often had as many as 75% of their patients presenting with both major mental illness and severe substance abuse problems. Similarly, the Progress Foundation acute alternatives were the first 24-hour psychiatric programs to treat acutely ill patients who were HIV positive or who had AIDS. Even the inpatient unit placed such individuals on medical wards with psychiatric consultation. The acute alternatives serve as an entry point to the system. If they maintain a policy of admitting all referrals, they will be the early warning alarm for any new complicating problems in the public mental health population.

This challenge to remain flexible is one of the most difficult principles to maintain in public systems of care. It demands a special kind of staff who are comfortable with ambiguity and experienced with innovative solutions to unanticipated problems. For this reason, Progress Foundation stresses an attitude rather than a manual of policies and procedures when training staff. Although manuals have their place in all programs, it is critical to the success of the acute alternatives that staff learn how to analyze situations and how to generate solutions on the spot. In any acute or crisis program, the ability to improvise on a theme is much more critical than the ability to memorize a tune.

Willingness to take risks. The treatment or service principles outlined in this chapter cannot be implemented unless the host organization, from the board of directors to the line staff, is willing to take risks. Many mental health programs become stultified and, ultimately, irrelevant because the management and staff have become too conservative in their approach to services. Risk-avoidance policies, fear of litigation, and an increasing climate of regulation in the field all contribute to this situation. In fact, if the Progress Foundation programs had been proposed in the current atmosphere regarding risk and innovation, it is doubtful that our agency would have had the opportunity to demonstrate the effectiveness of acute residential treatment.

Every time mental health programs propose a rule or institute a new procedure in the interest of minimizing risk, we must recognize that we also limit the opportunity for patients to demonstrate capability and learn the limits of their abilities. Rules and procedures are necessary in all services, and Progress Foundation has its share, but they must be used judiciously because they can stifle the very growth and change that is at the cornerstone of our programmatic ethic and intent. In a sense, every rule or procedure should pass a type of "environmental impact study" to assess its necessity and its effect on the rehabilitation goals of the program.

Shortly after Progress Foundation opened its third acute alternative—Cortland House—the staff wanted to meet with me to discuss their proposal to require a weapons search before admission to the program. Individuals, about whom very little was known, were being referred from the emergency room. Other patients and staff had raised questions of their own personal safety because some of the more acute patients were holding weapons among their personal belongings. Progress Foundation had never instituted a search procedure before. In two full staff discussions, we reviewed the necessity for the procedure, attempted to assess whether it would actually prevent the problem or just make staff and patients feel better, and assessed the impact of such a procedure on a social model, community program.

The result was that Cortland House implemented a search procedure as a part of admission to the program. However, it took a specifically social model twist in that the procedure was to ask each new patient if he or she had anything in their possession that could be considered a weapon. We found that patients voluntarily surrender a variety of weapons, ranging from handguns, in more than one instance, to a large machete. It was a rule and a procedure that was necessary in an urban, highly stressed community mental health system. The solution grew from discussions with staff and patients and was mindful of the necessity to guard the character and nature of the program.

The willingness to take risks, of course, extends to the basic premise of providing acute residential treatment services. Each time an individual in an acute episode is diverted to a community residence, a risk is created, regardless of how well staffed and experienced that community residential program may be. If the community program attempts to provide a noninstitutional environment that is as normalizing as possible, then the potential risk is increased. This risk, however, is not a clinical risk. It is a political and legal risk. The clinical efficacy of acute residential treatment programs has been demonstrated for almost 2 decades. Progress Foundation's acute programs have diverted approximately 10,000 individuals over the past 18 years, and there have been no incidents in the community. Fewer than 9% of those men and women who have been admitted over the years have been hospitalized from the acute programs, when we were unable to stabilize the acute episode. However, if an incident should occur in the community, we understand that the methods, practice, and policy of diverting individuals will come under close scrutiny. In fact, one unfortunate circumstance could close the program despite this record of success over the years. The agency must be willing to accept this risk in order to provide an effective program.

Within the program itself, this willingness to take risks extends to the commitment to maintain as normal a household environment as possible. This means that patients can come and go without signing in or out. Some individuals may be on a "close watch" status in the house, and, therefore, their movements are monitored. However, this status for one person does not have to extend to everyone. Similarly, a house setting provides opportunities for individuals to avoid contact or hide from staff. Rather than design an environment that places everyone in a setting that provides ongoing monitoring, the acute programs place the responsibility on each patient to communicate with staff and to control his or her impulses.

The Progress Foundation programs practice awareness rather than surveillance. Over the 18 years and 10,000 individuals treated by the acute programs, we have experienced fewer than a dozen violent episodes. This record is not due to any unusual ability of the emergency room or the acute program staff to discern the potentially violent patient from others. In fact, referrals to the acute houses are determined more by the availability, or lack of availability, of inpatient beds than by any particular set of uniform standards. The lack of violence in the Progress Foundation residential programs is directly attributable to the fact that our staff are with patients all the time. The programs are small, home-like environments in which staff and patients interact on a continual basis. Staff members know what is going on with all patients and are able to intervene early in an escalating crisis to avoid confrontations and potential violence.

Although there is not a great deal of visible, traditional structure, in the sense of rules, regulations, and physical design, there is a complex structure based on human interaction and awareness. There is also a sense of relaxation and safety that tends to de-escalate tense situations. Staff are trained to mediate and support, rather than to enforce or demand. The program stresses the point that individuals who may have been violent in one situation will not necessarily be violent in another, particularly if the environment is nonconfrontational.

Recently, one of the acute programs admitted a young woman who had managed to set fire to a seclusion room in the psychiatric emergency services while she was in four-point restraints. When she arrived at the acute program, she said that she would not repeat the fire-setting behavior in the house because she "was mad at the doctors in the hospital, but she was not mad at La Posada." She completed her stay in the residential setting very successfully and without incident.

The risks that any agency takes are not blind risks. Each risk, in terms of program design or patient freedom of movement, for instance, is calculated and strategic. In fact, risk management is a crucial element of the Progress Foundation programs. But for us, risk management means understanding and monitoring risk so that we can take maximum advantage of the potential of our patients, staff, and environments. It does not mean risk limitation. This principle requires constant review and vigilance because, with the willingness to take risks goes the responsibility to ensure that those risks are well considered and calculated so that the patients, the community, and the agency are not put in jeopardy.

Conclusion

The five principles outlined above form the ideological underpinnings of the Progress Foundation acute diversion services. It is the hope of the agency that they represent dynamic goals for the organization and staff, at all levels. The principles guide the implementation of a constantly shifting acute residential treatment program that provides a normalizing environment for the development of daily living skills, learning and testing of interpersonal skills, and individual growth and development.

The residential setting encourages and supports the efforts of patients to learn, or relearn, essential skills of daily living, such as personal hygiene, shopping for healthy food, cooking, maintaining a clean household, and surviving on a limited budget. This skill training is a critical aspect of both the crisis stabilization effort and the longer-term rehabilitation goals of the acute programs.

In addition, the acute residential programs are social-relational environments in which patients interact with one another, and with staff, in order to learn, develop, and test the complicated skills of interpersonal relationships.

When I first began work as a counselor in the first Progress House in 1969, patients would tell me that they wanted to learn "how to get to know people" in the program. Today, the single most frequently cited reason that patients identify as a factor in their psychiatric crisis is "loneliness." Whatever biochemical or social origin of the phenomenon of mental illness that we are attempting to treat, one thing has not changed in 2 decades: we are treating alienation and loneliness.

Residential treatment environments that are human-scale and "user-friendly" offer the opportunity to address the social aspect of recovery from severe mental illness. The environments bring people together and provide a context for individuals who have been alienated from their peer group, and their culture, to interact and find positive ways of living with other people. The acute phase of a crisis is a particularly dynamic opportunity to reinforce interaction with others, rather than to isolate and separate the individual experiencing the crisis from others.

Finally, acute residential treatment offers an opportunity to provide one-to-one counseling, support, and encouragement to patients. The small, interpersonal environments allow patients to discuss their dreams, their plans, their joys, and their sorrows with a sympathetic ear.

In fact, one of the major skills required of all staff in an acute alternative is the ability to listen. It has become popular in the public mental health field to describe those with severe and persistent mental illness as individuals who are not amenable to talk therapy. Increasingly, over the years, "therapy" for the patients has consisted primarily of pharmacological interventions. It has been my experience, throughout my career, that the patients in our programs have always wanted to talk. They may not conform to the system expectation that they talk in certain groups, or at certain times in a therapist's office, but they will talk if we are willing to listen. Some of the most successful connections between counselors and patients are made in our acute houses late into the night, sitting around the dining room table, or on a walk around the neighborhood. If we encourage them to talk, if we offer an environment of trust and responsiveness, and if we are willing to listen—to attend— rather than to dictate, diagnose, or intervene, then we begin to learn about each individual patient as a person with a unique life and a unique soul.

In many ways, attending to the safety and growth of each individual soul, to the best of our ability, is our primary task.

Acute work, particularly in urban communities, demands an ability to move quickly, change directions, and improvise solutions in rapidly changing circumstances. Progress Foundation has developed acute residential treatment programs that embody these qualities. The programs utilize the principles and practices of residential treatment, along with crisis intervention techniques and approaches and a strong community orientation, to produce acute programs that are noninstitutional, cost-effective, responsive to systemic demands, and grounded in an ethic that stresses dignity, respect, and self-determination for patients of the public mental health system.

Chapter 5

Northwest Evaluation and Treatment Center, Seattle: Alternative to Hospitalization for Involuntarily Detained Patients

Editor's Note

THE TREATMENT FACILITY DESCRIBED IN THIS CHAPTER, NORTHWEST Evaluation and Treatment Center, is an alternative to psychiatric hospital care that defies most of the principles of acute residential treatment outlined in the previous chapter. It is a large, locked, nondomestic facility with ambulance entrances and large elevators to accommodate patients strapped to gurneys: it does not aim to involve the resident in maintaining or shaping his or her living environment. Out of concern that the facility would be viewed as "not a hospital," the staff have gone to lengths to emphasize the medical nature of the program. It is designed for the evaluation of involuntary patients and has three secure rooms and clearly defined institutional operating procedures. Patients progress through a four-level system of privileges based on staff assessment. As a locked facility, the program is not integrated into the community. People cannot do the things they would normally do; instead, they are involved in recreational, art, and movement therapy.

This unit is essentially similar to a traditional psychiatric hospital unit, but is not licensed as such and is not as expensive as a hospital ward. The program is included here to illustrate the breadth of possibilities encompassed by the term *hospital alternative.*

Northwest Evaluation and Treatment Center, Seattle: Alternative to Hospitalization for Involuntarily Detained Patients

William D. Ferguson, M.D.
Daniel Dowd

*N*orthwest Evaluation and Treatment Center (NWETC) is a private, locked psychiatric facility in the state of Washington under contract to the King County Department of Human Resources. The unit serves patients who are involuntarily detained according the criteria set forth in the Washington State administrative code (Regulatory Code of Washington 71.05, Washington Administrative Code 275-55). It serves the greater Seattle area, with a population of approximately 1.5 million, and works with adults who have been committed for short-term acute treatment for periods of 72 hours to 14 days. Although NWETC is similar to a traditional psychiatric unit, its origins and licensure are different. It is an alternative to inpatient hospital treatment for acute involuntary psychiatric patients.

History of the Development of Evaluation and Treatment Centers in Washington State

Between 1980 and 1981, Washington State experienced a 90% surge in the number of involuntary psychiatric hospitalizations and thereby resultant costs. This phenomenon primarily resulted from the expansion of the involuntary commitment categories from "danger to self" and "danger to others" to include a new category defined as "grave disability" (Regulatory Code of Washington 71.05).

In the state of Washington the grounds for detention (Annotated Revised Code of Washington 1994) are

- Danger to self—"a substantial risk that physical harm will be inflicted by an individual upon his own person, as evidenced by threats or attempts to commit suicide or inflict physical harm on one's self" (p. 4).
- Danger to others—"a substantial risk that physical harm will be inflicted by an individual upon another, as evidenced by behavior which has caused such harm or which places another person or persons in reasonable fear of sustaining such harm" (p. 4).
- Danger to property—"a substantial risk that physical harm will be inflicted by an individual upon the property of others, as evidenced by behavior which has caused substantial loss or damage to the property of others" (p. 4).
- Grave disability—"a condition in which a person, as a result of a mental disorder, a) is in danger of serious physical harm resulting from a failure to provide for his own essential human needs of health or safety, or b) manifests severe deterioration in routine functioning evidenced by repeated and escalating loss of cognitive or volitional control over his or her actions and is not receiving such care as is essential for his or her health or safety" (p. 4).

Within 2 years of the addition of the grave disability category, the number of detentions to hospital beds in the Seattle area grew from approximately 1,000 people per year to 1,900 people per year. The state's hospital resources were strained, and the local psychiatric units in general hospitals expressed reluctance to increase their services to involuntary psychiatric patients. The Washington State legislature responded to this crisis by assigning the state division of mental health the task of finding alternative means of treating this segment of the population.

Part of the solution to this problem was to create a new licensing category known as adult residential treatment facility (Washington Administrative Code 248-25). The authorization of these facilities allowed for the development of local, specialized programs and avoided the certificate of need process. The challenge was to create facilities and programs that could respond to the intensive needs of this acute population in freestanding, nonhospital settings. These facilities would come to be known as evaluation and treatment centers, or E&Ts, and are monitored by both state and county agencies in Washington.

The initial attempt at development of an E&T failed in 1982. In September 1983, the first E&T was opened. The need was so great and the first model proved to be so successful that the principles involved in its creation were used to set up a second E&T; in August 1984, NWETC was opened. It is the focus of this chapter.

The Commitment Process in Washington State

The detention and commitment laws in the state of Washington are very close to the model adopted by the National Institute of Mental Health (Figure 5–1). All requests for evaluation for detention in King County are referred to the King County Crisis and Commitment Services Office. The office is staffed with county-designated mental health professionals (CDMHPs) who are nonphysicians and who are exclusively authorized in Washington to evaluate detention for a probable cause. The CDMHPs conduct an in-person interview to determine whether grounds for detention are present. Detention is based on the CDMHPs' evaluation of two factors: the presence of a mental disorder, and, as a result, the determination that the person is a danger to self, others, property, or is gravely disabled. The initial detention for a probable cause is 72 hours.

During this initial 72-hour period, the detained patient receives a comprehensive psychiatric and physical examination, as well as an evaluation by a forensic psychologist or psychiatrist for the purpose of court testimony. At the probable cause hearing after 72 hours, if the patient is found to still have a mental disorder and there are grounds for detention, he or she can be committed for up to an additional 14 days. This may be followed by additional 90- and 180-day commitment periods, with judicial review occurring at each juncture (Figure 5–2).

Issues in the Development of Evaluation and Treatment Centers

The initial attempt to set up an E&T failed in 1982 because of concerns by the nursing staff that the facility was not medically safe. When we began setting up NWETC, concerns were raised by the local medical community about the safety of this nonhospital facility. The following is a discussion of the major concerns expressed at the start-up of NWETC, how the concerns were addressed, and a description of the program.

First Issue: Patient Selection

What type of patient could not be treated in this setting?

It was determined early in the planning phase that exclusionary criteria must be narrow and highly specific for NWETC to function as a viable alternative to local and state hospitals, but we needed to be able to treat medically ill patients as well as those who were potentially aggressive. The availability of seclusion and restraint would be necessary. On-site pharmacy, laboratory, and primary care medical services would also be needed to treat patients with a wide range of presenting problems.

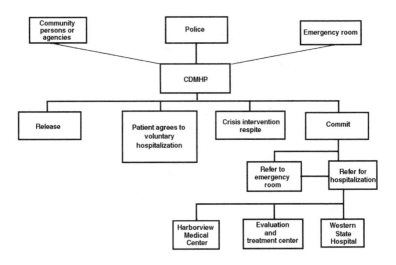

Figure 5–1.   Commitment procedures in Washington State. CDMHP = county-designated mental health professional.

Exclusionary criteria at the start-up were defined as:

1. Patient is less than 18 years of age.
2. Patient is nonambulatory (defined as inability to transfer self from wheelchair to bed or toilet).
3. Patient is medically compromised (having a condition that would be best treated in a hospital setting).

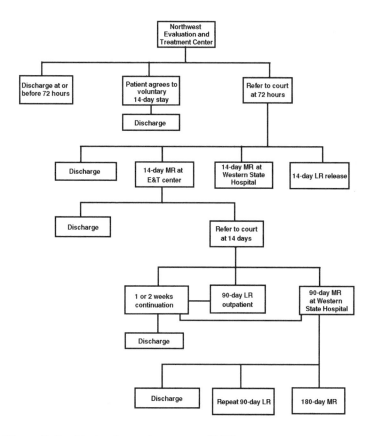

Figure 5–2. Evaluation and treatment (E&T) center options. MR = more restrictive court order (inpatient); LR = lesser restrictive court order (outpatient).

4. Patient is a felon (requiring 24-hour armed guard).
5. Patient is showing symptoms of organic brain syndrome and has never been worked up.

All patients who did not fall into one of the five exclusionary categories were to be admitted. If there was a question about the medically compromised nature of a patient, they were to be evaluated in an emergency room prior to admission. Criterion 5 was later removed from the exclusionary criteria list because it proved to be impossible to determine by a telephone screening process whether a patient had been "worked up."

For aggressive patients, three seclusion rooms were designed according to Washington administrative code specifications (WAC 248-18). A certified instructor in "nonoffensive methods of controlling aggressive behavior" was hired, and this person developed written unit procedures and a staff training program. All staff had to demonstrate proficiency in working with patients with aggressive behavior during probation and annually as a condition of employment, to be determined through written tests and physical demonstration.

Contracts were established with a local pharmacy providing on-site pharmacy services, delivery of medications, and consultation by a registered pharmacist. A local laboratory provided phlebotomists, specimen pickup, and testing with critical values established by NWETC. A contract was established with a community health center to provide physician assistant services on a daily basis, supervised by an internist.

By providing for these needs, NWETC was able to ensure treatment to all but significantly medically compromised or extremely violent patients.

Second Issue: Screening Process

How could we prevent the admission of patients requiring a higher level of care than the center could provide?

To review the patient's need for treatment, a telephone screening procedure was developed. The CDMHPs evaluate the patient and convey the information necessary for admission to the intake screener at the receiving facility. This information includes events prior to admission, psychiatric history, medical history, drug and alcohol involvement, physical handicaps, medical concerns, mental disorders and grounds for detention, and current level of behavioral control. The telephone screening lasts 7 to 10 minutes, and all screeners are trained individually by the program director. Before they begin telephone screenings, prospective screeners must accompany the CDMHPs in the field during a routine workday to observe commitments and interventions so that the screeners understand the need for prompt and timely responses to admission requests by the CDMHPs.

Third Issue: Referral Process

If a medically compromised or aggressively dangerous patient was admitted to the unit, could we recognize and treat, or transfer, these patients in an appropriate, timely manner?

In order to address these concerns several agreements and collateral contracts were negotiated. These agreements included the following:

- NWETC would be able to transfer to Harborview Medical Center (HMC), the county hospital 1 mile away, patients who were either medically compromised on arrival at the unit or who became medically compromised during their stay at NWETC.
- NWETC would be able to transfer to the HMC maximum security psychiatric ward patients who became behaviorally unmanageable when the seclusion rooms were unavailable, or when NWETC staff believed that a behavior management transfer was necessary on therapeutic grounds (i.e., following a staff injury, or after one patient injured another).
- NWETC would be able to send patients for medical workups and assessments to the HMC emergency room or clinics either prior to accepting a patient for admission or during a patient's stay at NWETC.

We consulted with the head of the emergency physician's association for the state of Washington. He advised against the administration of intravenous medication or fluids or any more invasive procedures and advocated for training the staff in cardiopulmonary resuscitation (CPR) and for using the local 911 emergency team for acute medical emergencies. All staff are trained in CPR as a condition of employment, and any patient requiring intravenous medication or fluids is transferred to the HMC emergency room. For acute medical emergencies, we call the 911 medical emergency team. The response time of the medical emergency team is 3 to 5 minutes.

Evaluation and Treatment Process

Once we had satisfied ourselves that we were able to screen out or refer inappropriate patients, we turned to the issues of the design of the evaluation and treatment process.

The E&T is different from voluntary psychiatric hospitals because there is a court evaluation on all patients at the end of 72 hours and after 14 days. Each patient has an attorney, and the court decides whether a patient must stay beyond 72 hours or 14 days. We had specific legally mandated time lines (24 hours, 72 hours, and 14 days) and needed to design a process that would incorporate these time lines and the court evaluations.

24 hours. A comprehensive evaluation is completed within the first 24 hours of admission. This process includes

- A medical assessment performed by admitting staff to detect acute emergencies.
- A physical examination completed within 24 hours of admission by the physician assistant or the psychiatrist. Additional consultation from a community health center or HMC is obtained if necessary. Vital signs are routinely monitored twice daily for all patients for 2 days unless more frequent monitoring is indicated.
- A psychiatric evaluation performed by the psychiatrist on duty. This includes a mental status examination, a psychosocial history, and an initial DSM-IV (American Psychiatric Association 1994) diagnosis. Any treatment deemed necessary is initiated. For a nighttime admission, the psychiatrist is called and the patient is described over the phone. Initial orders are given by phone, and the psychiatric examination commences the next morning. If the staff believe that the patient is having acute medical problems on admission, they will call the psychiatrist and then either call 911 or send the patient to the HMC emergency room by ambulance.

- A complete battery of blood tests done on a routine basis. Laboratories provide 24-hour turnaround on routine tests, and emergency laboratory services are also available, if necessary. ECGs are done on the ward as needed. X rays, computed tomography (CT) scans, and other tests are done when necessary at HMC.

72 hours. In addition to the above, during the first 72 hours on the unit the patient receives

- Daily evaluations by mental health professional staff members to determine whether both a mental disorder and grounds for detention persist.
- A psychological evaluation by a forensic psychologist to determine whether to petition the court for further hospitalization beyond the 72-hour period. The psychologist will testify at this hearing if it is determined necessary to petition for one.
- An extensive psychosocial evaluation, which begins with the admission process, incorporates the patient's psychosocial history data taken by the psychiatrist, and is completed by the treatment coordinator assigned to the case. Informants for these data might include the patient, family and friends, outpatient psychiatric and medical sources, and previous hospital records.

14 days. During the 14-day period

- A treatment coordinator is available on each shift for every patient.
- Psychiatric and medical problems are treated as necessary.
- A psychiatrist evaluates each patient at least every 4 days, or sooner if indicated.
- The patient's condition is discussed daily by staff in a consultation group.
- A forensic psychologist performs an evaluation before the final discharge is implemented. If a longer hospitalization is necessary, at another hospital, this information is conveyed to the court.

These procedures were then integrated into the overall program design. Evaluation and treatment, although stated as two discreet processes, are interrelated and progress simultaneously.

Program Design

NWETC began with the following goals and objectives:

- To provide a safe, structured environment in which involuntarily detained patients can regain stability
- To maintain a clean, pleasant, well-organized milieu that stresses adaptive skills while diminishing symptoms and maladaptive behaviors
- To ensure goal-directed planning of interventions utilizing methods that stress dignity and patient choice
- To formulate realistic treatment goals for short-term stay
- To maximize continuity of care for patients by implementing a treatment and discharge planning process that is individual, flexible, and comprehensive
- To maintain accessibility to all individuals and agencies who may be part of the support and treatment network
- To provide a local cost-effective alternative for involuntarily detained patients to minimize disruption of their lives, and to reinforce continued relationships with families, support systems, and service providers
- To provide timely and useful data with a context of collaborative planning to community treatment agencies to ensure coordinated assessment and treatment
- To become an integral link between Western State Hospital and local residential facilities for recalcitrant patients

We have designed a program around these goals. NWETC is an acute, short-term psychiatric facility with an average length of stay for patients of 14 days. The basic treatment modalities are psychopharmacology as well as individual reality orientation and support provided in the context of a caring environment. As described for other brief hospitalizations, stabilization of the patient, crisis intervention, and discharge planning are emphasized (Sederer 1992).

Milieu meetings are held twice a day (and as necessary) to address ward dynamics and interactions. Recreational, art, and movement therapies are used throughout the week. Staff members assigned to each patient provide individual therapy, which generally focuses on reality-oriented issues. There is a four-level system; patients move up the levels and acquire greater privileges based on staff assessment (in consultation group) of each patient's progress.

Each shift is supervised by a team leader, and the average ratio of staff to patients is 1:5. The daily clinical operation is supervised by a clinical director (Table 5–1).

NWETC employs four psychiatrists, each of whom works in 24-hour segments. The psychiatrist assumes responsibility for all 32 patients when he or she begins work at 8 A.M. Psychiatrists work on the unit for 8 hours; the first priority is to do psychiatric evaluations on new admissions. The unit averages two admissions per day, but we have accepted as many as seven patients in a 24-hour period. This task is followed by evaluations of difficult or problem patients. These patients are identified in the A.M. shift change, and the physician is informed. Other tasks for the psychiatrists include 4-day reviews of all patients (patients are seen at least every 4 days by the psychiatrist), privilege level increases, discharge orders, and leave orders. When the psychiatrist leaves the unit, he or she continues to accept calls for the remainder of the 24-hour period, and then turns over the entire patient population to the psychiatrist who begins duty at 8 A.M. the next day. Such a system requires a high level of communication between the psychiatrists, which occurs on a daily basis as well as at twice-monthly meetings of psychiatrists and the program director.

Physician assistants are on the unit daily to perform physical examinations and to provide continued care for patients with physical problems such as diabetes and hypertension. The physician assistants are supervised by an internist from their agency and consult on a daily basis with the NWETC psychiatrists. The psychiatrist performs these duties on weekends. Interpreter services, art and movement therapy, and maintenance are also provided.

The unit staffs to a 26-hour day (two 8-hour shifts and one 10-hour shift), thus allowing a 2-hour shift overlap daily between the day and

Table 5–1.   Clinical supervision

Program director	1
Clinical director	1
Forensic psychologist	1
Discharge supervisor	1
Psychiatrists	4

evening shifts. The expense involved is justified by the clinical benefit of having the time to adequately discuss the cases with the maximum number of clinical participants present (Table 5–2). With this level of staffing, we have been able to adequately meet our goals and legal time lines to evaluate and treat the patients while providing a warm supportive environment.

The treatment plan, which is our central tool for this evaluation and treatment process, is individualized and problem oriented. It focuses initially on the immediate needs before concentrating on short-term needs and, finally, longer-term goals. Treatment plans are reviewed daily by the treatment coordinators assigned to the patient and are reviewed in daily consultation groups in the presence of all treatment staff. Treatment goals for each patient are discussed on a daily basis.

The implementation of a discharge plan is an active process involving the patient, the discharge coordinator, and outside service providers or resources. The discharge coordinator reviews all choices available to the patient and allows the patient, as much as is feasible, to make the choices that fit his or her particular needs and preferences.

On discharge, all agencies receive a packet containing information on the patient's stay at NWETC, including treatment plan, psychosocial data, medications, and medical information. This information maximizes the opportunity for continuous patient care.

Table 5–2.   Direct care staff

	#Staff/ day shift	#Staff/ evening shift	#Staff/ night shift
Team leader	1	1	1
Psychiatric nurse	2	2	1
Mental health professional	1	1	1
Mental health specialists	4	4	2
Recreation specialist	1	1	
Unit secretary	1	1	
Court transportation	1		
Patient services coordinator	1		
Discharge planner	1		

Discussion

NWETC has been open since 1984 and has treated 600 patients per year. After 8 years, our experience with a nonhospital acute psychiatric unit has taught us that it is a feasible, cost-saving method of treating involuntarily detained, mentally ill patients. There are very few involuntarily detained patients who cannot be treated in this type of unit. Because of the fear that we are "not a hospital" or "not medical enough," we have gone to great lengths to emphasize the medical components of this facility. Because we have had the cooperation of community-oriented agencies, such as community health centers, HMC, and the county medical emergency team (911), we have been able to treat patients with all but the most acute medical problems that most physicians would recognize as requiring hospital care (e.g., myocardial infarction or cerebrovascular accident). Most "minor" medical problems can be treated on the unit by our medical team. Occasionally, we have had to transfer patients to HMC because we could not control them behaviorally. These were usually patients diagnosed with antisocial personality disorder with polysubstance abuse who were seeking drugs, and we did not have available seclusion rooms. On several occasions, patients have injured staff members, and we believed that it would be best to transfer the patient to another unit for therapeutic reasons.

In general, our patients are a younger population (average age of 37.5 years). Three percent of our patients have been over age 65, with a greater likelihood of medical problems. We have been able to effectively treat this elderly population, if the medical problems have not been acute emergencies and did not require intravenous medication or fluids.

We have used all the standard psychiatric medications for this severely disturbed population, and patients have had the usual side effects. We tend to avoid the use of respiratory-depressing medications, but the use of lorazepam in conjunction with neuroleptics appears to have decreased the overall doses of neuroleptics necessary to control very agitated patients. This is also perhaps why we have avoided the more dangerous side effects of the neuroleptics (e.g., neuroleptic malignant syndrome, acute laryngospasm).

As Table 5–3 shows, we have seen patients from a range of diagnostic categories. In addition, substance abuse and Axis II diagno-

Table 5–3.   Diagnostic groupings

Schizophrenia	29%
Bipolar affective disorder	21%
Major depression	19%
Atypical psychosis	12%
Organic affective disorder	8%
Adjustment disorder with depression	4%
Schizoaffective disorder	3%
Miscellaneous	4%

ses are made in 50% of our patients. We have been able to return approximately 70% of the patients to local treatment and living situations (Table 5–4). The 10% of patients transferred to the state hospital usually have been schizophrenic patients refractory to traditional neuroleptics and patients with difficult personality disorders. We have been able to meet our goal of keeping the majority of patients close to their support and treatment networks. Approximately 14% of patients have had to be transferred to other hospitals for medical or behavioral reasons or for inpatient alcohol or substance abuse treatment.

The E&T concept appears to be a cost-saving alternative to a hospital setting. The daily bed rate is $230. The average cost per patient stay at an E&T is approximately one-third of the cost per stay in a traditional hospital psychiatric unit (Table 5–5). A county-owned building that is architecturally suited for this type of facility (e.g., ambulance entrances, large elevators that can accommodate gurneys) is

Table 5–4.   Discharge plans (7/89 to 6/90)

Return to former residence	42%
Transfer to state hospital	10%
Medical transfer, voluntary hospitalization, inpatient alcohol treatment, behavioral transfer	14%
New living situation (e.g., congregate care facility, semi-independent living situation)	34%

Table 5–5. Average cost per stay: evaluation and treatment centers (E&Ts) versus hospitals

E&Ts	1,300 patients per year × $230/day × 14-day LOS = $4,186,000/year
	Average cost per patient stay = $3,220
Local hospitals	1,300 patients per year × $700/day × 14-day LOS = $12,740,000/year
	Average cost per patient stay = $9,800

Note. LOS = length of stay.

used. The E&Ts in the county average 90% occupancy and a 14-day length of stay.

Conclusion

There are now four E&T facilities in the state of Washington, and more are in the planning phase. Recent Washington State law has mandated that by July 1, 1993, 85% of persons who are detained or committed for up to 17 days must be treated in the local regional support network (Washington Administrative Code 275-56, Senate Bill 5400, 1989). This will likely increase the need for more E&T facilities or similar forms of treatment for acutely ill committed psychiatric patients. This type of facility is similar to the psychiatric health facilities in California and will likely become more popular in other states as the concept of treating chronically ill psychiatric patients close to their support network becomes more popular and the competition for mental health monies increases (Moltzen et al. 1986).

References

American Psychiatric Association: Diagnostic and Statistical Manual of Mental Disorders, 4th Edition. Washington, DC, American Psychiatric Association, 1994

Annotated Revised Code of Washington, Vol 16, Section 71.05.020. Charlottesville, VA, Michie Company Law Publishers, 1994, pp 4–6

Moltzen S, Gurevitz H, Rappaport M, et al: The psychiatric health facility: an alternative for acute inpatient treatment in a nonhospital setting. Hosp Community Psychiatry 37:1131–1135, 1986

Sederer LI: Brief hospitalization, in American Psychiatric Press Review of Psychiatry, Vol 11. Edited by Tasman A, Riba MB. Washington, DC, American Psychiatric Press, 1992, pp 518–534

Chapter 6

Acute Hospital Alternatives in the Netherlands: Crisis Intervention Centers

Editor's Note

CRISIS INTERVENTION CENTERS WERE ORIGINALLY DEVELOPED IN THE Netherlands in response to the theoretical approach outlined by Caplan (1963) in his *Principles of Preventive Psychiatry.* The original goal of providing preventive intervention to previously healthy people under severe stress did not prove feasible, but the crisis centers proved their value in other ways, developing into short-term treatment units for more chronically disturbed people. Seven of these short-term residential facilities are in operation in the Netherlands. The author describes three programs, in Groningen, The Hague, and Rotterdam—important components of the Dutch mental health system functioning as alternatives to hospital treatment for a wide range of psychiatrically disturbed people.

Acute Hospital Alternatives in the Netherlands: Crisis Intervention Centers

Willem J. Schudel, M.D., Ph.D.

*I*n this chapter, I describe the development and operation of community-based crisis centers in the Netherlands, which provide acute residential care and treatment for patients with a variety of social and psychiatric problems.

The Residential Care of Psychiatric Patients in the Netherlands

The Netherlands is a small, densely populated country with approximately 15 million inhabitants as of 1993. The population has increased by 2 million since 1970. The country has an extensive network of health care facilities. Historically, the general practitioner (GP) has fulfilled a central role by providing primary health care and referring general and mental health problems to appropriate institutions. At present, there is one GP for every 2,300 inhabitants.

The mental health system mainly comprises

- General psychiatric hospitals
- Various categories of psychiatric hospitals (including those for drug addiction, forensic psychiatry, and juvenile psychiatry)
- Psychiatric wards of general hospitals
- Regional institutions for outpatient mental health care (community mental health centers)
- Psychogeriatric nursing homes
- Psychiatrists in general practice

In addition, over the years, various experimental and permanent intermediate care clinical and psychosocial programs have been established. Examples of these include the so-called multifunctional units and the psychiatric and psychosocial crisis centers. At these facilities, outreach services are offered in addition to short-term psychiatric care.

The scope of residential care for psychiatric patients in the Netherlands did not change as dramatically after the Second World War as it did, for example, in the United States and in the United Kingdom. Because the quality of care provided at psychiatric hospitals was generally of high standard, and treatment concerns prevailed over purely custodial functions, compulsory closures or reductions in the size of the hospitals were not necessary. The older hospitals were modernized, however, and decentralization encouraged the dispersal of institutional beds. In fact, in the Netherlands only a few very large psychiatric hospitals exist, with a capacity of 1,000 to 1,500 beds.

The criteria for residential treatment in the Netherlands have differed from Anglo-Saxon psychiatry over the years, as well as today. In the Netherlands, the majority (approximately 85%) of patients admitted to psychiatric hospitals are admitted voluntarily. It is not only seriously psychotic or dangerous patients who are admitted, but also those with neurotic disorders, moderately severe depression, and personality disorders. Psychotherapy is still an important part of treatment at all residential psychiatric institutions. The broad intake criteria are responsible for the large number of available psychiatric beds and admissions to psychiatric hospitals. In 1990, the number of psychiatric hospital admissions was 2.34 per 1,000 inhabitants. The primary diagnosis was schizophrenia in only 12.7% of admissions, and psychosis was suspected in fewer than 50% of patients.

For many years, 1.5 beds per 1,000 inhabitants have been available at general psychiatric hospitals in the Netherlands. The total cost of mental health care in 1991 was estimated at ƒ 6 billion (U.S. $3 billion), of which about 80% was spent on residential care in hospitals and nursing homes, and 13% was spent on outpatient care, including psychiatrists in general practice and psychotherapists (NcGv 1993).

Despite the liberal availability of residential treatment facilities, there were waiting lists for admission in many places in the early 1970s. The pressure this exerted on hospitals and outpatient facilities led to a discussion of alternative reception facilities and, finally, to the development of crisis intervention centers.

The Birth of Crisis Intervention Centers

In the Netherlands, as early as the 1930s, Querido in Amsterdam, among others, conducted pioneering work in the field of social psychiatry. After the war, the interest for preventive activities grew strongly as a result of the international focus on the Mental Health Movement. In 1963, Caplan published the book *Principles of Preventive Psychiatry,* in which he elaborated further on Lindemann's (1944) classic crisis theory. Caplan's book was particularly well received in the Netherlands and rapidly formed the basis for new mental health policy. Under the new policy, professional aid was made more accessible to people in social or psychological crisis who did not show signs of full-blown psychiatric disorder. By bringing such aid closer to the public and demonstrating its effectiveness, an attempt was made (in line with Lindemann's and Caplan's theories) to use the crisis situation for therapeutic purposes and to begin a process of reintegration of the affected individual. This resulted in a distinction, for theoretical reasons, between unexpected crises ("life events") and developmental crises, which are a part of normal human life (Erikson 1968). Weathering a crisis successfully, with or without external aid, may lead to a new balance at a higher level of integration. An unsuccessful crisis intervention, or the absence of adequate aid, may lead to an actual psychiatric presentation (e.g., depression or psychosis).

Since 1970, a number of small facilities specifically directed toward intensive, short-term crisis intervention were established, particularly in the large cities. These facilities were experimental and remained so for a long time, largely because most of them had unorthodox financing. Most of the crisis centers had a full professional staff, consisting of physicians, psychologists, social workers, and nurses. The facilities were staffed according to the usual standards in force at the time. The goals of the crisis intervention center required that it be accessible to new patients during the day and night; in addition, a combination of beds and outpatient services, unusual for that period of time, were available at most of the centers. If all the beds at a center were occupied, services would be available to new patients, even though they could not be admitted. One of the earliest centers took crisis theory very literally by assigning employees on each shift to every patient. They worked, as it were, in an uninterrupted shift system on the crisis of the involved patient. Each of the centers retained its own style of providing aid, although the common denominator of their therapeutic approach was to prevent admission to regular psychiatric hospitals.

This approach attracted financing by health insurers who were prepared to pay the relatively high daily charges per patient based on the fact that the majority of patients would return home to receive subsequent guidance and counseling from their GP or from an outpatient service. At most of the centers, duration of admission was restricted by health insurers—usually to 7 or 10 days. If the patient required a longer stay, permission had to be obtained for the case in question. After 1983, because of government restrictions, most of the centers were assigned to provide either psychosocial assistance or psychiatric crisis intervention. Rotterdam is one of the few examples where both forms of aid (and financing) coexist.

In general, centers were successful in maintaining rapid turnover and short duration of stay. Some centers accepted only patients referred by GPs, whereas others accepted anyone who walked in on their own accord to request aid. The crisis intervention centers were located in a variety of settings. Most centers formed a part of a general or academic hospital; a few were established as independent operating units in the city.

Developments Since 1970

During the 1970s, an awareness gradually developed that Caplan's crisis theory was not a panacea for setbacks in life. After the initial optimism, crisis intervention staff were confronted more often with cases of "relapsing crisis." These involved individuals with a susceptible personality disposition and/or a disturbed social background who decompensated easily under stress and who repeatedly requested aid. "Real" cases of crisis, that is, in otherwise healthy and balanced individuals who decompensated temporarily because of severe stress, appeared to be rare. The availability of this primary target group was temporarily increased only after disasters, such as large multiple traffic accidents or kidnapping. In the Netherlands, crisis care for healthy individuals who have experienced a severe trauma has been increasingly left to voluntary aid workers, because it appears that, in most of these cases, professional attention is not required. There are now victim assistance agencies throughout the country. Therefore, over time, most of the crisis centers have admitted a considerable number of "permanent" patients. The need for temporary intervention (time-out) for chronic patients in distress has been noted by, among others, Hoult (1986) in Sydney, Australia, and Stein (1992) in Madison, Wisconsin (Stein and Test 1980). However, crisis intervention has not been abandoned. It remains useful, despite changes in the population served, to provide short-term, intensive intervention to prevent long-term hospital admission.

A second change occurred in the 1980s. In 1981, regional institutions for outpatient mental health care (RIAGGs) were created by law. These institutions, to a certain extent comparable with the American community mental health centers (CMHCs), were given regional responsibilities, including the obligation to provide acute psychiatric care 24 hours a day, 7 days per week (7×24-hour service) in their catchment area. For most of the crisis centers, this meant a closer cooperation with the RIAGG in their region and a restriction of direct access for the public and the primary care providers.

Patients with acute mental health problems are referred to the 7×24-hour service by the GP. If necessary, this service calls in the crisis center. It is of interest, however, that the extension of acute outpatient care in the Netherlands has *not* decreased the pressure on the residential facilities. On the contrary, in most areas it is more difficult now to admit an acute psychiatric patient (e.g., a patient with schizophrenic psychosis) to a psychiatric hospital than it was before 1980. Apparently, this is a result of administrative problems within the psychiatric hospital rather than an actual problem with capacity. The increased pressure for residential care may also be attributed to a "tip of the iceberg" effect: the increased availability of psychiatric care in the community has probably stimulated requests for such aid. The number of individuals who request aid at the RIAGGs has increased yearly, although there is barely any indication that the Dutch population as a whole is under greater mental stress.

The crisis centers have retained their place and function within the changing structure of mental health care. New centers are rare, but existing centers are extremely busy—partly, in the classical sense, as an alternative to hospital admission, and partly as a buffer for the overcrowding in mental health facilities that continues despite increased capacity.

Seven existing, operational crisis centers (with a capacity varying from 7 to 12 beds) totally or partially focus on intensive, short-term care for acute psychiatric patients. In addition, numerous centers in the Netherlands offer psychosocial assistance to homeless people, battered women, runaway juveniles, and others who are not registered as patients of the health care system. In the following sections, I describe in detail three crisis centers that differ from each other in various aspects.

Unification in Diversity: Three Examples

Groningen

Groningen, with a population of 170,000, is the capital city of a moderately large province in the northern part of the Netherlands. The crisis center is part of the university psychiatric clinic, which is located within the boundaries of the academic hospital. It has 10 beds and opened in 1971 as one of the first centers.

Staff.   The staff comprises 14 nurses, 2 psychiatric residents (one of whom is assigned to training in consultation-liaison psychiatry), and 1 social worker/family therapist. A psychotherapist (nonmedical) coordinates the center, but a part-time senior psychiatrist has ultimate medical responsibility. The majority of the staff have served at the center for many years. At least two nurses are present in the facility during the day and night. The admission staff at the psychiatric clinic initially evaluate requests for admission. Admission criteria are very broad, but, because the unit is open and has no special detention facilities, seriously psychotic and dangerous individuals are not admitted. The outside door of the unit is closed at night for security reasons, but patients can be admitted 24 hours a day. The center has single rooms, double rooms, and a room that accommodates three people.

Program.   A nurse and, usually, a physician conduct an intake interview to compile a thorough inventory of the patient's problems. This inventory is completed within the following 48 hours, after which a counseling plan is prepared. The purpose of the counseling plan is to restore the premorbid balance as soon as possible so that the patient can be transferred to the regular outpatient service (i.e., the RIAGG or the GP). Team meetings are held twice a day to evaluate and adjust, if necessary, the counseling plans for all patients. The therapy includes a wide array of possible interventions, such as medication and short-term psychotherapy (individual or system oriented). In practice, almost 60% of the patients return home after approximately 1 week.

Although the center is located within the psychiatric hospital department, it is run like a household. Patients set the table, make their own beds, and may leave the building for shopping or other activities if they inform the staff.

Statistics.   An average of 350 individuals are admitted to the center each year. The average duration of admission has gradually increased from 4.5 days in 1973 to 8.7 days in 1988. Sometimes, one or two patients stay a month or longer. Approximately two-thirds of those admitted are women; this proportion has increased over the past 10 years. One-quarter of the patients are referred by physicians in the emergency wards of the academic hospital; almost all are people who have attempted suicide. Nearly 20% are referred by psychiatrists in the nearby outpatient department, and about 15% are in treatment with GPs and RIAGGs. Eight percent of the patients are self-referred. Almost 75% of the patients are from the city of Groningen or its immediate vicinity.

Diagnosis.   Almost 25% of the patients appeared to be psychotic on admission, approximately 15% had a depressive syndrome without psychotic features, and 7% had a substance use diagnosis. In 30% of patients there was no DSM-III-R (American Psychiatric Association 1987) Axis I diagnosis. There was evidence of personality disorder in almost one-third of patients. More than one-half of all patients had previously been admitted to a psychiatric hospital.

After discharge from the crisis center, 60% of the patients went home, 30% were transferred to the university psychiatric clinic, and 10% were admitted to other nonpsychiatric institutions or homes.

Cost.   Admission to the center for a maximum of 3 weeks is reimbursed by AWBZ (General Health Insurance Act). The all-inclusive cost per person per day is *f* 601 (U.S. $300). A single episode of treatment of average duration (8.7 days) thus costs *f* 5,228 (U.S. $2,614). The total annual cost of the crisis center to the community is approximately *f* 1,800,000 (U.S. $900,000).

Summary. The crisis center in Groningen has a clear psychiatric signature that has become even clearer through the years. The majority of the patients, in fact, are psychiatrically ill and have often relapsed. Adjustment disorders (e.g., as a result of a serious, emotionally traumatic experience) in premorbidly healthy, balanced individuals are seldom observed. The center functions mainly as an intermediate care facility to prepare patients for adequate outpatient or hospital treatment. Nevertheless, it seems likely that many patients who return home after spending time at the crisis center would have been directly admitted to a psychiatric hospital in the absence of the crisis center. From this point of view, the original goals of the center, namely, preventing admission to a psychiatric hospital, have been successfully met.

The Hague

The Hague is the third largest city in the Netherlands. It has a population of 450,000 and is the parliamentary seat of the Dutch government. The crisis intervention center has 10 beds and was set up in the early 1970s in a property purchased in the inner city. Over the past few years, the center has cooperated extensively with the urban 7×24-hour psychiatric service provided collectively by the three RIAGGs in The Hague. The nurses at the center participate in the 7×24-hour service.

The staff comprises 1 part-time psychiatrist, 1 resident, 1 part-time GP, 1 social worker, and 18 nurses. One GP in training is also regularly employed at the center. At least two nurses are present at the center during the day and night. Maximum stay at the center is 8 days, by agreement with the regional health insurers. Only in exceptional cases is permission granted to retain a patient for more than 8 days.

On admission to the center, the staff attempt to solve the patient's presenting problems and to refer the patient for further outpatient treatment. These problems range from psychosocial issues to serious psychiatric disorders. Sometimes problems are so complex that admission to a psychiatric hospital is indicated. The center also acts as a buffer by temporarily receiving patients who have been referred for admission to a psychiatric hospital that has no current vacancies. Thus, the center fulfills the following tasks: time-out or respite care, observation and diagnosis, crisis intervention with the aim of keeping the patient functional, and holding and preparing the patient for admission to a psychiatric hospital.

Referral to a psychiatric hospital always occurs via the RIAGG. A psychiatrist or a resident evaluates the need for admission. Somatic problems are investigated before admission and systematically recorded.

Program. Immediately after arrival, an extensive inventory of all possible psychosocial and psychiatric problems is commenced. Whenever possible, a psychiatric diagnosis is established, and treatment is initiated. The acquaintances (family, friends, and employer) of the patient are involved in compiling the inventory and, if required, in tackling the problems. Directed short-term psychotherapeutic intervention is the rule because it is necessary to strictly adhere to restrictions in duration of stay. The psychiatrist is ultimately responsible for all therapy. Because the center is located downtown, patients go out shopping and visit other agencies. Most patients do household chores and join each other at meals and at leisure time.

Statistics. Through the years, there has been a great deal of consistency in the type of patients admitted. More women than men were admitted (in 1989, 59% were women). The age group of 25–45 years is overrepresented by comparison with the general population of The Hague. There are 500 to 550 admissions annually (in 1989, 535 admissions). Almost 75% of the patients came from The Hague, and most of the remainder came from the immediate vicinity. All referrals came from professionals at RIAGGs. One-third of the patients who were admitted to the crisis center were readmissions.

In 1989, 23% of all the patients admitted were transferred to a psychiatric hospital. In about 40% of the patients in this group, the admission had been previously planned. About 65% of those requesting aid returned home after staying at the center, and 5% went to other health care facilities.

Diagnosis. On admission in 1989, 23% of the patients were psychotic, 18% had a depressive syndrome without psychotic features, and 14% had a substance use diagnosis. In 13% of the patients, the criteria for an Axis I diagnosis were not met. A personality disorder was reported in 10% of the patients at discharge. Almost one-third of those requesting aid had been previously admitted to the crisis center, one-half of them within the previous year.

Cost. The all-inclusive charge to the AWBZ (national health insurance fund) amounts to ƒ 730 (U.S. $365) per person per day. An average stay of 5.4 days costs almost ƒ 4,000 (U.S. $2,000). Total annual costs for the program are ƒ 2.2 million (U.S. $1.1 million).

Summary. The crisis center in The Hague focuses on observation, diagnosis, and short-term crisis intervention for individuals with slight to moderate psychopathology. The severity of the crisis and the intensity of the treatment vary a great deal. The "local color" of the center is fundamentally different from that of the admission ward at a psychiatric hospital. This is apparent from the limited number of patients who are transferred to the psychiatric hospital, beyond those who were temporarily held while awaiting a vacancy at the hospital. As mentioned earlier, the center fulfills an important function as a holding area when hospitals are at capacity.

Rotterdam

Rotterdam is the second largest city in the Netherlands and the largest seaport: it has more than 1 million inhabitants. The crisis center in Rotterdam opened in 1979 and is established in a large, old mansion near the city center. In 1988, a second crisis center in the southern part of the city (on the opposite bank of the river) was opened. The crisis centers in Rotterdam are not financed by the health insurers on the basis of episodes of treatment: they are jointly funded by the health insurers and the municipal authorities. The center in Rotterdam-South is not included in the account presented here.

The crisis center in central Rotterdam operates in cooperation with the regional psychiatric hospital and the RIAGGs. The center has 12 beds—6 are reserved for patients with social problems and 6 for psychiatric crisis intervention. These 6 psychiatric beds are available to the 7 × 24-hour service of the RIAGGs. A clear distinction is made between the counseling and treatment of psychiatric and psychosocial patients.

The center is open during the day and night and accessible to those in distress and in need of assistance. At night, two staff members are present (as a rule, a psychiatric nurse and a social worker). The accommodations consist of single rooms, double rooms, and a room for receiving an entire family. The crisis center also serves as a base for the

7 × 24-hour outreach service. Members of the general public in Rotterdam can request aid at the crisis center themselves or by referral. Help is available to all those in acute psychosocial or psychiatric distress. Every patient is interviewed and screened for admission according to a limited number of selection criteria. As a rule, aggressive patients and those addicted to drugs are referred to other facilities that are better equipped to deal with them. The same applies to the long-term homeless people who need shelter. The aim of the crisis center is to analyze the acuity of distress, to prevent it from escalating, and to help restore the balance between the individual's coping strength and level of stress. The center strives to provide additional outpatient care to as many patients as possible.

The staff comprises 24 permanent members (18.6 full-time equivalents [FTEs]), 8 substitutes, and 1 or 2 part-time on-call psychiatrists. Psychiatry is the only distinct discipline (0.5 FTEs). The remainder of the staff have different backgrounds and qualifications. The nurses and social workers are registered as crisis intervention employees and provide primary care in the urban 7 × 24-hour service, where a psychiatrist is also on call.

Program.   The center offers a safe environment for the patient to calm down. Interviews are conducted to compile an inventory of problems and to find possible solutions. Medication is provided when necessary, and the patient is encouraged to reestablish contact with those who have previously provided help. The duration of stay is restricted to a maximum of 6 days. This center has the most casual atmosphere of the three described in this chapter. Patients come and go freely for shopping in the downtown neighborhood, and they assist in running the household as if they all were part of an extended family.

Statistics.   In 1991, there were 490 admissions to the psychosocial beds and 365 admissions to the psychiatric beds. There were 378 episodes of outpatient intervention for psychosocial patients and 365 outpatient interventions for psychiatric patients. The average duration of admission for the center as a whole was only 2.35 days. Almost 50% of all the psychiatric patients had been admitted to a psychiatric hospital in the past. Approximately 60% of those requesting aid were women (70% of those with psychosocial problems and 53% of those with psychiatric problems). About one-third of the patients were self-referred, almost 15% were referred by professionals at the RIAGGs, and 12% were referred by the police.

Diagnosis.   The annual report of the crisis center does not include information on diagnoses; it only includes the primary stress that led the individual to contact the center. The most frequently cited sources of stress in 1990 were threats and abuse, 20% (30% of female patients); relationship problems, 17% (20% of women); and depression, including 12% who had attempted suicide. It is important to note that 58% of the women who sought aid did not return home; most went to a shelter for battered women. Thirteen percent of those who requested aid were referred to a psychiatric hospital.

Cost.   The average cost per intervention (there are almost 1,600 crisis interventions per year) is ƒ 950 (U.S. $475). The total annual cost of the crisis center is estimated at ƒ 1,500,000 (U.S. $750,000).

Summary.   The crisis center in Rotterdam has a very broad target group. The duration of stay at this center is very short. Every day, three or four new patients (with social or psychiatric problems) receive assistance. Psychiatric patients are either treated very quickly or are referred. A holding function (because hospital beds are full) is almost unnecessary in Rotterdam because of the extensive cooperation between all of the social and medical facilities. Everyone knows about the center, and the staff can quickly arrange other types of assistance. The center serves as a backup for a large number of other facilities in the city. In comparison with other facilities, the ample staffing pattern at the center enables it to provide intensive aid quickly.

Conclusion

The crisis intervention centers have won an important position as alternatives to acute psychiatric hospital care, especially in the large Dutch cities. The centers have limited capacity but, because of rapid turnover, are almost always able to admit new patients. The rapid turnover is due to synergy among the following factors:

- A relatively large professional staff with extensive experience
- An exchange of personnel with the 7 × 24-hour service that provides

the acute psychiatric care for the community
- A good arrangement with psychiatric hospitals for quick transfers
- Excellent, often personal, contacts with all the relevant medical and social service institutions (including the police, social services, and various reception centers)
- A financial system of Dutch health care in which the costs are never a hindering factor for those requesting aid

A cost-benefit analysis is required to evaluate whether public funds used in this manner are well spent. As yet, such an analysis of Dutch health care is not available. The operational costs of the centers are not particularly modest, but because no real cost-benefit analysis is available, the regional health insurers are willing to meet the costs. This willingness may be related to the fact that, in the Netherlands, there are no procedures limiting the duration of stay at psychiatric hospitals. A system such as the United States' diagnostic related groups (DRGs), in which only a limited duration of stay is reimbursed by the health insurers, has not yet been implemented here. In the Netherlands, a routine first-time admission to a psychiatric hospital for observation, diagnosis, and treatment of a patient with acute psychosis often takes 6 weeks. Because nursing charges average f 300 (U.S. $150) per day, such a routine short-term admission costs the health insurers a total of f 5,400 (U.S. $2,700). Taking this into account, admission-preventing interventions, such as those provided at the crisis centers, are relatively inexpensive. At various locations throughout the country, other experiments in outpatient care aimed at preventing hospital admission have been conducted. To date, these have not led to a generally acceptable system that can be used on a large scale.

Even so, it is remarkable that, since 1980, the number of crisis centers has not grown beyond the small group of institutions that already existed. At present, therefore, one can only speak of a useful and accepted alternative to acute psychiatric care, but not of the solution. It is likely that the crisis centers are seen as nonstigmatizing by the general public and referring authorities. Although this question has not been explored extensively, it appears that those who request assistance are largely satisfied with the help provided and would be willing to return in the future if necessary. Further investigations are important for an effective assessment of the value and the efficacy of the crisis centers in cases of psychiatric distress.

References

American Psychiatric Association: Diagnostic and Statistical Manual of Mental Disorders, 3rd Edition, Revised. Washington, DC, American Psychiatric Association, 1987

Caplan G: Principles of Preventive Psychiatry. New York, Basic Books, 1963

Erikson E: Identity: Youth and Crisis. New York, WW Norton, 1968

Hoult J: Community care of the acute mentally ill. Br J Psychiatry 149:137–144, 1986

Lindemann E: Symptomatology and management of acute grief. Am J Psychiatry 101:141–148, 1944

NcGv (Nederlands Centrum voor Geestelijke Volksgezondheid: Dutch National Institute for Mental Health): Geestelijke Volksgezondheid szorgingetallen, 1993

Stein LI: Crisis stabilization services for persons with psychotic illnesses, in Emergency Psychiatry Today. Edited by Van Luyn JB, Rijnders CATh, Vergouwen HHP, et al. Amsterdam, Elsevier, 1992, pp 25–28

Stein LI, Test MA: Alternatives to mental hospital treatment, I: conceptual model, treatment program and clinical evaluation. Arch Gen Psychiatry 37:392–397, 1980

Part II

Innovative and Nontraditional Programs

Editor's Note

SOTERIA IS A DESCENDENT OF KINGSLEY HALL, A NOVEL NONMEDICAL community for people with psychosis, which radical British psychiatrists R. D. Laing and David Cooper helped to develop in London in the 1960s. Soteria and its sister program, Emanon, were small supportive households established in California in the 1970s to provide care for people with first-episode schizophrenia, using minimal amounts of antipsychotic medication. A controlled investigation, funded by the National Institute of Mental Health and reported here by the project founder, Loren Mosher, demonstrates that psychosocial care in this type of therapeutic milieu produces results that are equivalent to or better than standard hospital and outpatient treatment—at no greater cost and without reliance on usual doses of neuroleptic medication.

Chapter 7

The Soteria Project: The First-Generation American Alternatives to Psychiatric Hospitalization

Loren R. Mosher, M.D.

*I*n the spring of 1971, a two-story, 12-room, 1912-vintage, wooden house on a busy thoroughfare in San Jose, California, became the first in a series of successors to Kingsley Hall, the London-based residential alternative to hospitalization started by the Philadelphia Association in 1965. (R. D. Laing and David Cooper were its best known members.) True to its heritage, Soteria House (Figure 7–1) was in the midst of a multiethnic working-class neighborhood. However, it had a number of advantages over its East London parent. First, substantial numbers of college students and former state hospital patients lived in this desig-nated poverty area. Hence, transience and deviance were not unknown. Second, painting the exterior of the house and replanting its rundown yard helped us win acceptance in the community. Third, my London experience convinced me that the house and its staff should attempt to conform to neighborhood social norms. In contrast, the community surrounding Kingsley Hall was instrumental in closing it. Fourth, there were explicit rules prohibiting certain behaviors—suicide, violence, unannounced visitors, and sexual relations between staff and patients. Fifth, because there was a paid staff, attention to life's necessities was ensured.

Into this comfortable six-bedroom home came—for 3 to 6

Portions of this chapter appeared previously in "Soteria: A Therapeutic Community for Psychotic Persons." International Journal of Therapeutic Communities 12:53–67, 1991. Those portions are reprinted here with permission.

months—an unusual group: young, unmarried people newly diagnosed and labeled as having schizophrenia. Six people could be accommodated at any one time. Another somewhat less unusual group—the nonprofessional staff—also lived there to provide a simple, homelike, safe, warm, supportive, unhurried, tolerant, and nonintrusive social environment. Soteria staff believed that sincere human involvement and understanding were critical to healing interactions with patients. The purpose of this project was to determine whether this type of milieu was as effective in promoting recovery from mental illness as that provided in a nearby general hospital's psychiatric ward, where the most valued treatment was antipsychotic drugs.

Four years later, a second house, Emanon, opened. The intention was to provide an immediate replication of the original milieu in a new community with different staff and leadership, but with the same research design. Ordinarily, the patients at Soteria House (and later at Emanon) received no antipsychotic drugs for 6 weeks after entry. The staff believed that it might take that long before important relationships could form and before the special qualities of the culture there could be meaningfully transmitted. The original facility, Soteria House, closed

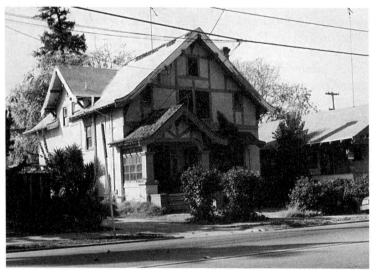

Figure 7–1.   Soteria House, San Jose, California.

in November 1983. Emanon House closed at the end of 1980. Both closures were the result of the end of research grant funding. Data analysis was not completed until March 1992.

Background

Although my experiences at Kingsley Hall were important to the development of the Soteria Project, difficulties in treating patients with psychosis in hospital settings also provided a major impetus for the type of facility that was developed—a home where schizophrenic patients who would otherwise have been hospitalized lived through their psychosis with a nonprofessional staff. Hospitals—even well-staffed "progressive" ones—invariably have institutional characteristics that create barriers to establishing the types of relationships that could maximally facilitate the process of recovery from psychosis. The "barrier" characteristics (present to varying degrees in different settings) are described in the following sections.

Theoretical Model

Most psychiatric wards function primarily within a medical model. Doctors have final authority and decision-making powers; medications are accorded primary therapeutic value and are used extensively; patients are seen as having a disease, with attendant disability and dysfunction that is to be "treated" and "cured"; and labeling and its consequences, objectification and stigmatization, are almost inevitable.

In contrast, at Soteria (from the Greek, salvation or deliverance) the primary focus was on growth, development, and learning. The staff were to "be with" the patients, or residents as they were called, to facilitate these processes. Decision-making powers and responsibility were shared with the residents. The staff were not there to "treat" or "cure" the residents. Although the medical model has demonstrated heuristic value, its application to patients with psychiatric disorders has unfortunate (and unintended) consequences for individual patients. No alternative model was proposed, however, and none seemed to satisfactorily explain the label "schizophrenia." Instead, an alternative "attitude," "stance," or "view" was proposed: an interpersonal phenomenologic approach to schizophrenia, that is, an attempt to understand and share the psychotic person's experience, and one's reactions to it, without judging, labeling, derogating, or invalidating it.

Size

Most psychiatric hospital wards have at least 20 patients. Thus, the staff-to-patient ratio is apt to be 40:60. For severely disorganized persons, however, it is important for the social reference group to have no more than 12 to 15 persons. A group of this size, when combined with a homelike atmosphere, maximizes the possibility for a disorganized person to become familiar with and to trust a new environment and to find a surrogate family in it, while it minimizes the labeling and stigmatization process. It is interesting that this is approximately the maximum number of patients able to live under one roof as an extended family or commune. In addition, most clinicians believe that 12 patients is the upper limit for effective group therapy. Finally, the small task groups in experimental psychology have been shown to function best with no more than 12 members. Thus, rather than a 20-bed ward, Soteria and Emanon were homes where 8 to 10 slept comfortably, with six beds occupied by residents and two by staff.

Social Structure

Social structure interacts closely with size; to function effectively, every organization, large or small, needs structure. In general, the larger the organization, the greater the structure. Unfortunately, more elaborate structures have hierarchy-related consequences that interfere negatively with psychotic persons. Inflexibility, reliance on authority, institutionalization of roles, and decision-making power and responsibility residing in the hierarchy are outside patients' control. Inevitably, those at the bottom of the hierarchy feel powerless, irresponsible, and dependent. As a result, Soteria was as unstructured as commensurate with adequate function. Structure that developed to meet functional needs was dissolved if the need did not continue. There was no institutionalized method of dealing with a particular occurrence. For example, overt aggressive acts were handled in various ways, including physical control (but not seclusion, straitjackets, or forced medication), depending on many contextual variables.

Medication

We live in an overmedicated, too frequently drug-dependent culture. We resolve our ambivalence about drugs by creating two categories:

good drugs (e.g., alcohol) and bad drugs (e.g., lysergic acid diethyl-amide [LSD]). Psychiatrists' attitudes are no different from that of the wider social context; the magical answer is sought from a pill. The antipsychotic drugs have provided psychiatrists with real substance for their magical cure fantasy with regard to schizophrenia. As is the case with most such exaggerated expectations, the fantasy is better than the reality. After nearly four decades, it is clear that the antipsychotic drugs do not *cure* schizophrenia. Antipsychotic drugs also have serious, sometimes irreversible, toxicities (Crane 1973), they may impair recovery in at least some patients with schizophrenia (Goldstein 1970; Rappaport et al. 1978), and they have little effect on long-term psychosocial adjustment (Niskanen and Achte 1972). This is not to deny their extraordinary use in reducing and controlling symptoms, shortening hospital stays, and revitalizing interest in schizophrenia.

One aim of the Soteria Project was to seek a viable, informed alternative to the overuse of, and excessive reliance on, these drugs—often to the exclusion of psychosocial measures. We used them infrequently, and, when prescribed, they were kept primarily under the individual resident's (patient's) control. That is, we asked the resident to monitor his or her response to the drug carefully and to give us feedback so we could adjust the dosage. After a trial period of 2 weeks, the resident largely influenced the decision of whether to continue the drug.

The Soteria Project was a reaction to criticisms of existing facilities in each of the four areas that are mentioned above. However, a good deal of what was involved in the program was based on the positive contributions of other researchers, clinicians, and theorists. In fact, we realized that no individual element of the Soteria program was new; we believe that it was the combination into one setting that was unique.

Soteria's roots include the era of moral treatment in America (Bockoven 1963), the tradition of intensive interpersonal intervention in schizophrenia (Fromm-Reichmann 1948; Sullivan 1962), therapists who have described growth from psychosis (Menninger 1959; Perry 1962), the group of psychiatric heretics (Laing 1967; Szasz 1961), and descriptions of the development of psychiatric disorders in response to life crisis (Brown and Birley 1968).

Research Design

Sample Selection

All subjects were from screening facilities that were part of the community mental health center (CMHC) complexes containing our control wards. Anyone who met the following basic criteria was a potential study candidate:

- Patients with symptoms clearly diagnosed as schizophrenia
- Patients who needed to be hospitalized
- Patients who were not previously hospitalized more than once for 4 weeks or less with a diagnosis of schizophrenia
- Patients who were ages 18–30 years (male or female)
- Patients who were unmarried, separated, widowed, or divorced

The selection criteria are designed to provide a relatively homogeneous sample of individuals with diagnoses of schizophrenia, who are also at risk for prolonged hospitalization or chronic disability. Early age at onset and being unmarried have both been shown to be predictive of the need for chronic care (Strauss et al. 1977).

Because of research grant–related changes (see "Treatment Assignment" below), patients treated at Soteria were divided into two cohorts: Cohort I, encompassing 1971–1976, and Cohort II, encompassing 1976–1983. Cohort I had 37 experimental and 42 control subjects, and Cohort II had 45 experimental and 55 control subjects. Cohort II included the subjects treated at Emanon.

Treatment Assignment

Subjects meeting study selection criteria were identified without knowledge of the group to which they would ultimately be assigned. Study requirements were explained, and informed consent was obtained from the patient and family, or significant other, if available. In the 1971–1976 study cohort, because of limited experimental bed availability, subjects were assigned on a consecutively admitted, space-available basis to Soteria House. Subjects in the 1976–1983 cohort were assigned on a strictly random basis to Soteria or Emanon.

Research Assessment

Below is a partial list of the measures completed at baseline (admission to the study) and at follow-up (6 weeks, and 6, 12, and 24 months postadmission). All assessments were conducted by an independent research team that had no direct treatment responsibilities in either setting.

- **Baseline**
  Diagnosis—As per DSM-II (American Psychiatric Association 1968). Three independent diagnoses of schizophrenia must be in agreement for inclusion in the study.
  Diagnostic symptoms—A checklist of seven symptoms. Four of seven symptoms are required for inclusion in the study (Cole et al. 1964).
  Certainty of diagnosis—A 7-point scale (Mosher et al. 1971).
  Mode of onset—Assesses acute- or insidious-onset types (Vaillant 1964).
  Paranoid or nonparanoid status—A short scale for rating paranoid schizophrenia (Venables and O'Connor 1959).
  Global severity—An overall measure of psychopathology.
  Brief social history form—A detailed description of a patient's and family's psychiatric and social history (Boothe et al. 1972).
- **Follow-up**
  Patient progress report—For each 6-month interval, information was obtained on the subject's medication history, other treatments used, living arrangements (including any hospital readmissions), work status, social contacts, global severity, and improvement.

Clinical Settings

Experimental

Soteria was a 12-room house located on a busy street in a "transitional" neighborhood of a San Francisco Bay Area city. Bordering Soteria on one side was a nursing home and on the other, a two-family home. Emanon was a very similar house, but it was located in a somewhat quieter neighborhood. It was surrounded by other similar homes.

Based primarily on licensing laws, each house could accommodate only six residents at one time, although as many as 10 persons could sleep there comfortably. There were six paid nonprofessional staff, a house director, and a quarter-time project psychiatrist at each facility. One or two new residents were admitted each month. In general, two of our specially trained nonprofessional staff, a man and a woman, were on duty at any one time. In addition, at least one volunteer was present, especially in the evening. Most staff worked 36- to 48-hour shifts to enable them to relate to "spaced-out" (their term) residents continuously over a relatively long period of time. Staff and residents shared responsibility for household maintenance, meal preparation, and cleanup. People who were not "together" were not expected to do an equal share of the work. Over the long term, staff did more than their share and would step in to assume responsibility if a resident could not do a task to which they had agreed. The house director was friend, counselor, supervisor, and object for displaced angry feelings by staff. The part-time project psychiatrists supervised the staff and were seen as stable, reassuring presences (in addition to their formal medicolegal responsibilities).

Although staff varied somewhat in how they saw their roles, they generally viewed what psychiatry labels a "schizophrenic reaction" as an altered state of consciousness in an individual who was experiencing a crisis in living. Simply put, the altered state involves personality fragmentation, with the loss of a sense of self.

Few clinicians would disagree with a description of the evolution of psychosis as a process of fragmentation and disintegration. But, in this project, the disruptive psychotic experience was also believed to have unique potential for reintegration and reconstitution if it was not prematurely aborted or forced into some psychologically straitjacketing compromise. This was very much in keeping with the ethos at Kingsley Hall. Such a view of schizophrenia implies a number of therapeutic attitudes. Soteria House staff members considered all facets of the psychotic experience to be "real." They viewed the experiential and behavioral attitudes associated with the psychosis—the clinical symptoms, including irrationality, terror, and mystical experiences—as extremes of basic human qualities. Because "irrational" behavior and mystical beliefs were regarded as valid and as capable of being understood, Soteria staff tried to provide an atmosphere that would facilitate integration of the psychosis into the continuity of the individual's life. Thus, psychotic persons were not to be considered "diseased," nor were they to be related to in a depersonalized way, because that would invalidate the experience. When the fragmentation process is seen as valid and as having potential for psychological growth, the individual experiencing the schizophrenic reaction could be tolerated, lived with, related to, and validated, but not "treated" or used to fulfill staff therapeutic ambitions. Limits were set if the person was clearly a danger to himself, others, or the program as a whole—not merely because others were unable to tolerate his or her madness. Antipsychotic drugs were ordinarily not used for 6 weeks. If the resident showed no change at that time, neuroleptic drugs were instituted at appropriate dosage levels.

Our rationale for the use of specially trained nonprofessionals as primary staff (see also Hirschfeld et al. 1977; Mosher et al. 1973) is that we believe that relatively untrained, psychologically unsophisticated people can relate to patients with psychosis more easily than highly trained professionals (e.g., M.D.'s or Ph.D.'s) can, because nonprofessionals have not learned a theory of schizophrenia, whether psychodynamic, organic, or a combination of both. Our nonprofessional staff members had the freedom to be themselves, to follow their visceral responses, and to be a "person" with the psychotic individual, because they did not have any preconceived ideas. Highly trained mental health professionals tend to lose this freedom in favor of a more cognitive, theory-based, learned response that may invalidate a patient's experience if the professional's theory-based behavior is not congruent with the patient's needs. Professionals may also use their theoretical knowledge defensively when confronted, in an unstructured setting, with anxiety-provoking behaviors of psychotic people. Our nonprofessional therapists tend not to respond in this manner.

CMHC Comparison Ward

The CMHCs' inpatient services consisted of two locked wards of 30 beds each. They were well-staffed (staff-to-patient ratio of 1.5:1) active treatment facilities oriented toward crisis intervention. High doses of neuroleptics were likely to be administered, and patients were quickly evaluated and placed in other parts of the treatment networks. All of the control patients reported here received antipsychotic drugs during their inpatient stays. Only one patient was discharged who was not taking drugs. The hospital staff members were generally well trained, experienced, and enthusiastic; they saw themselves as doing a good job.

Results

Cohort I (1971–1976)

Six-week and 2-year outcome data from the subjects admitted between 1971 and 1976 were reported in detail elsewhere (Matthews et al. 1979; Mosher and Menn 1978). Briefly summarized, the significant results from the initial, Soteria House only, cohort were

- *Admission characteristics*—Experimental and control subjects were remarkably similar on 10 demographic, 5 psychopathology, 7 prognostic, and 7 psychosocial preadmission (independent) variables.
- *Six-week outcome*—In terms of psychopathology, subjects in both groups improved significantly and comparably, despite Soteria subjects not having received neuroleptic drugs.
- *Milieu assessment*—Because we conceived the Soteria program as a recovery-facilitating social environment, systematic study and comparison with the CMHC were particularly important. We used Moos' Ward Atmosphere Scale (WAS) and COPES scale for this purpose (Moos 1974). The differences between the programs have been remarkable in their magnitude and stability over 10 years. As shown in Figure 7–2, the Soteria environment was perceived as significantly different from the CMHC milieu on 9 of 10 subscales of the Moos instrument. They were seen similarly on only the order and organization variable. This pattern remained stable (with minor fluctuations) for the project's 10-year life (Figures 7–3 and 7–4). COPES data from the experimental replication facility, Emanon, yielded a nearly superimposable figure. Thus, we concluded that the Soteria Project and CMHC environments were, in fact, very different, and the Soteria and Emanon milieus conformed closely to our predictions (Wendt et al. 1983).
- *Community adjustment*—Two psychopathology, three treatment, and seven psychosocial variables were analyzed. At 2 years postadmission, Soteria-treated subjects from the 1971–1976 cohort were working at significantly higher occupational levels, were more often living independently or with peers, and had fewer readmissions; 57% had never received a single dose of neuroleptic medication.
- *Cost*—In the first cohort, despite the large differences in lengths of stay during the initial admissions (about 1 month versus 5 months), the cost of the first 6 months of care for both groups was approximately $4,000.

Cohort II (1976–1982)

Admission, 6-week, and milieu assessments replicated almost exactly the findings of the initial cohort. However, in contrast to Cohort I, after 2 years, no significant differences existed between the experimental and control groups in symptom levels, treatment received (including medication and rehospitalization), or global good versus poor outcomes. Consistent with the psychosocial outcomes in Cohort I, Cohort II experimental subjects, as compared with control subjects, were more independent in their living arrangements after 2 years.

Interestingly, independent of treatment group, good or poor outcome is predicted by four measures of preadmission psychosocial competence: level of education (higher), precipitating events (present), living situation (independent), and work (successful) (L. R. Mosher, R. Vallone, A. Z. Menn, unpublished data, submitted to NIMH, March 1992). Good outcome was defined at both 1- and 2-year follow-up as having no more than mild symptoms *and* either living independently or working or going to school.

Conclusions

What have we learned from these two second-generation Kingsley Halls?

- Interpersonally based therapeutic milieus that are as effective as neuroleptic drug treatment in reducing the acute symptoms of psychosis in the short term (6 weeks) in newly diagnosed psychotic patients can be established and maintained.
- The therapeutic community personnel did not require extensive mental health training and experience to be effective in the experimental context. They did, however, need to be sure that this was the type of work they wanted to do, and to be psychologically strong, tolerant, flexible, positive, and enthusiastic. Finally, they needed good on-the-job training and easily accessible supervision and backup.
- Longer-term outcomes (2 years) for the experimental groups were as good as or better than those of the hospital-treated control subjects.
- It appears that the positive longer-term outcomes achieved by Cohort I, as compared with Cohort II experimental subjects, were at least partially a result of the spontaneous growth of easily accessible social networks around the facilities, although it is difficult to confirm this

from the data. These informal networks provided interpersonal support, housing, jobs, friends, and recreational activities on an as-needed basis to patients and staff. Unfortunately, these networks disintegrated once it became clear that the facilities would close. Hence, in contrast to Cohort I, Cohort II subjects did not receive much of the peer case management provided by the social networks around the houses during their 2-year follow-up.

System Change

Based on what I have presented in the "Research Design" and "Results" sections of this chapter, it is evident from the Soteria Project findings that newly diagnosed schizophrenic patients can be treated as well—or better—and at no greater cost in a nonhospital community setting as in a hospital. Our results are consistent with those of others who have studied nonhospital alternative treatments (e.g., Fairweather et al.

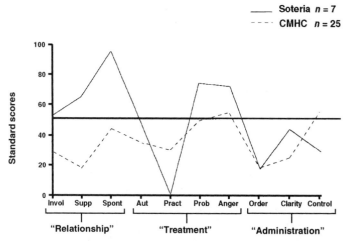

Figure 7–2. Comparison of Soteria staff and community mental health center (CMHC) staff using Ward Atmosphere Scale real testing based on staff norms for 160 wards. Invol = involvement, Supp = support, Spont = spontaneity, Aut = autonomy, Pract = practical orientation, Prob = personal problem orientation, Anger = anger and aggression, Order = order and organization, Clarity = program clarity, Control = staff control.

1969; Langsley et al. 1968; Pasamanick et al. 1967; Polak and Kirby 1976; Stein and Test 1976). In 19 of 20 studies, Straw (1982) found that outcomes were as good as or better in the alternative-treated groups compared with hospital-treated patients. Has this evidence resulted in a shift from the use of hospitals to the use of alternative methods of care in the United States? Basically, the answer is no.

Private practice–oriented psychiatrists in the United States have not been persuaded by the evidence that nonhospital alternatives are a useful ingredient in the therapeutic smorgasbord. However, in American public mental health, the notion of "crisis residences" has become popular (see Stroul 1987).

Why, in the era of so-called "scientific" psychiatry, have these types of facilities and clinical care paradigms not been widely implemented? The answer to this question is both complex and elusive. The most facile answer is that the studies were either insufficiently rigorous, did not provide convincing evidence, or were one-time, unreplicable products of the investigators' enthusiasm and dedication. As

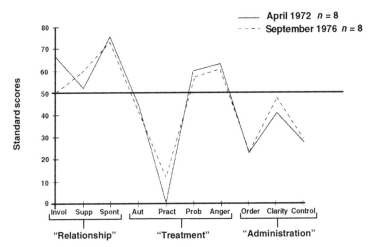

Figure 7–3. COPES change over time: Soteria staff. Invol = involvement, Supp = support, Spont = spontaneity, Aut = autonomy, Pract = practical orientation, Prob = personal problem orientation, Anger = anger and aggression, Order = order and organization, Clarity = program clarity, Control = staff control.

one of these enthusiastic investigators, I must ask how many comparative outcome studies of variations in hospital treatment are there?
Despite the vast numbers of patients hospitalized for psychiatric treatment each year (more than a million in the United States), there are very
few controlled outcome studies of systematically varied inpatient care
(Caffey et al. 1972; Glick et al. 1974; Herz et al. 1971). Although the
evidence supportive of the use of alternatives may not be incontrovert-
ible, there would appear to be more hard data relative to their usefulness
than there are for in-hospital treatment.

   If the evidence presented is in itself "acceptable," why is the next
step—its application to clinical care settings—not? I propose that the
implementation of alternatives is unacceptable because they represent
a threat to in-hospital psychiatry's turf. What elements of the Soteria
program (true to a greater or lesser extent for most alternatives) are

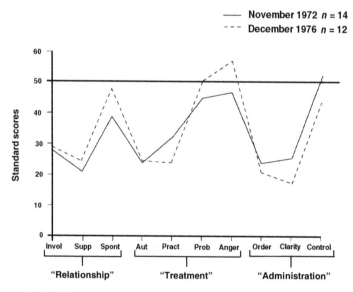

Figure 7–4.   Ward Atomosphere Scale change over time: Valley staff.
Invol = involvement, Supp = support, Spont = spontaneity, Aut = autonomy, Pract = practical orientation, Prob = personal problem orientation,
Anger = anger and aggression, Order = order and organization, Clarity
= program clarity, Control = staff control.

perceived as threats to hospital psychiatry?

In brief, the elements of the Soteria program most relevant to this discussion are as follows:

- The facility was not a hospital, and its program was not run by doctors or nurses by delegation. However, it admitted only patients who would have otherwise been hospitalized.
- Neuroleptics, the standard treatment for patients with schizophrenia, were used as infrequently as possible, preferably not at all.
- Primary treatment responsibility, power, and authority were vested in the nonprofessional staff.

How has traditional hospital psychiatry defended itself against this rather radical attempt to demedicalize psychosis? Four reasons seem most germane. First, foremost, and most effective, no third-party payers in the United States are willing to underwrite this form of care. This does not imply that psychiatry actively moved to prevent third-party payment for alternatives; rather only that it has not joined in to actively seek it.

The ultimate viability of alternatives in the therapeutic marketplace resides with funding sources—which is why they are becoming available in public systems but not private ones. How interested these fiscal intermediaries will be in paying for innovations in care is strongly influenced by the prevailing zeitgeist. In the last several decades there has been a substantial shift in American psychiatry's zeitgeist—away from a socioenvironmental one to a more medical biological point of view. Thus, there is little pressure from biomedically oriented mainstream psychiatry to pay for a basically nonmedical treatment. What are other relevant manifestations of the biomedical zeitgeist? It would appear that psychiatry is doing what it believes it must to continue to qualify for third-party payment (i.e., supporting hospital-based wards).

Second is the medicalization of community psychiatry—it is ironic that the now nearly 30-year-old community psychiatry movement in the United States has moved the mental health system back into closer juxtaposition with the somatic health system. That is, the relative isolation of mental health before the 1960s—as manifested in the state hospital systems—was broken down with the advent of community psychiatry with its emphasis on inpatient care on wards in general medical hospitals. The growth of such wards was also given impetus by psychiatric coverage in various health insurance programs and by government-sponsored medicare and medicaid. For the most part, payment for inpatient care in general hospitals has been the only consistently available mental health benefit. These two factors account in large part for growth of these wards and the increasing numbers of patients treated in them. For example, between 1967 and 1971, the numbers of schizophrenic patients treated in such wards nearly doubled—from 90,000 to 170,000 (Taube 1969, 1973).

This process of bringing "mental illness" back into the mainstream of medicine was given further impetus by numerous developments in medical technology. That is, an array of new, sophisticated techniques became available for use in the search for the "schizococcus" and other specific etiologies of mental illness. Application of these techniques to mental illness has provided us with a deluge of new information but has failed to discover specific etiologic factors in psychosis.

In addition, a new generation of technology-oriented biological psychiatrists has risen preferentially to positions of influence and power in many medical school departments of psychiatry.

The third important factor in the progressive medicalization of psychosis has been the introduction and widespread use of neuroleptic drugs—clearly efficacious treatment. Because drugs can only be prescribed by M.D.'s, as long as drugs are viewed as "the answer" to mental illness, doctors' power and control of the treatment system will increase. Because pills are given to individuals, they maintain medicine's traditional focus on a person as "diseased." This may prevent the doctor and the system over which he or she presides from looking at the family and wider social contextual factors that might have influenced the development of psychosis—and might also, therefore, be amenable to intervention. Thus, medications narrow conceptual sights and unnecessarily limit treatment possibilities.

The fourth is the waning influence of psychoanalysis. I believe it is fair to say that the 1950s and early 1960s were the heyday of psychoanalytic influence on more traditional psychiatry. Psychoanalysts and analytic theories were widely used for both descriptive and etiologic purposes. For a number of years it was almost de rigeur for residents in the best known training programs to enter analytic training.

In the late 1960s and through the 1970s their influence has been much diluted by waves of findings from the new technologists. The appeal of analytic constructs, so pervasive in the 1950s and 1960s, has been replaced by more reliably identifiable and quantifiable substances such as neurotransmitters and endorphins. Whether these high-technology findings have made a substantial contribution to clinical practice remains moot.

This evolution is complex in its derivation, but, nevertheless, psychoanalysis as a discipline does not seem to be as interested in psychosis as it was during its halcyon days. The neuroleptics, development of rapid turnover wards in general hospitals, and community psychiatry each contributed to what I perceive as a withdrawal of psychoanalysis's cathexis of psychosis.

References

American Psychiatric Association: Diagnostic and Statistical Manual of Mental Disorders, 2nd Edition. Washington, DC, American Psychiatric Association, 1968

Bockoven J: Moral Treatment in American Psychiatry. New York, Springer, 1963

Boothe H, Schooler N, Goldberg S: Brief social history for studies in schizophrenia: an announcement of a new data collection instrument. Psychopharmacol Bull 8:23–44, 1972

Brown GW, Birley JLT: Crisis and life changes and the onset of schizophrenia. J Health Soc Behav 9:203–214, 1968

Caffey EM, Galbrecht CR, Klett CJ: Brief hospitalization and aftercare in the treatment of schizophrenia. Arch Gen Psychiatry 24:81–86, 1972

Cole J, Klerman G, Goldberg S: Effectiveness of phenothiazine treatment in acute schizophrenics. Arch Gen Psychiatry 10:246–261, 1964

Crane G: Clinical psychopharmacology in its 20th year. Science 181:124–128, 1973

Fairweather G, Sanders D, Cressler D, et al: Community Life for the Mentally Ill: An Alternative to Institutional Care. Chicago, IL, Adline Publishing, 1969

Fromm-Reichmann F: Notes on the development of treatment of schizophrenia by psychoanalytic psychotherapy. Psychiatry 11:263–273, 1948

Glick I, Hargreaves WA, Goldfield MD: Short vs. long hospitalization: a controlled prospective study. Arch Gen Psychiatry 30:363–369, 1974

Goldstein M: Premorbid adjustment, paranoid status, and patterns of response to phenothiazine in acute schizophrenia. Schizophr Bull 3:24–37, 1970

Herz MI, Endicott J, Spitzer R, et al: Day vs. inpatient hospitalization. Am J Psychiatry 127:107–118, 1971

Hirschfeld R, Matthews S, Mosher LR, et al: Being with madness: personality characteristics of three treatment staffs. Hosp Community Psychiatry 28:267–273, 1977

Laing R: The Politics of Experience. New York, Ballantine Books, 1967

Langsley DG, Kaplan DM, Pittman FS, et al: The Treatment of Families in Crisis. New York, Grune & Stratton, 1968

Matthews SM, Roper MT, Mosher LR, et al: A non-neuroleptic treatment for schizophrenia: analysis of the two-year postdischarge risk of relapse. Schizophr Bull 5:322–333, 1979

Menninger K: Psychiatrist's World: The Selected Papers of Karl Menninger. Edited by Hall B. New York, Viking, 1959

Moos RH: Evaluating Treatment Environments: A Social Ecological Approach. New York, Wiley, 1974

Mosher L, Pollin W, Stabenau J: Identical twins discordant for schizophrenia: neurologic findings. Arch Gen Psychiatry 24:422–430, 1971

Mosher L, Reifman A, Menn A: Characteristics of nonprofessionals serving as primary therapists for acute schizophrenics. Hosp Community Psychiatry 24:391–395, 1973

Mosher LR, Menn A: Community residential treatment for schizophrenia: two-year followup data. Hosp Community Psychiatry 29:715–723, 1978

Niskanen P, Achte K: The Course and Prognosis of Schizophrenic Psychoses in Helsinki: A Comparative Study of First Admissions in 1950 (Monograph No 2). Helsinki, Psychiatric Clinic of the Helsinki University Central Hospital, 1972

Pasamanick B, Scarpitti FD, Dinitz S: Schizophrenics in the Community. New York, Appleton-Century-Crofts, 1967

Perry J: Reconstitutive process in the psychopathology of the self. Ann N Y Acad Sci 96:853–876, 1962

Polak PR, Kirby MW: A model to replace psychiatric hospitals. J Nerv Ment Dis 162:13–22, 1976

Rappaport M, Hopkins HK, Hall K, et al: Are there schizophrenics for whom drugs may be unnecessary or contraindicated? International Pharmacopsychiatry 13:100–111, 1978

Stein LI, Test MA: Training in community living: one year evaluation. Am J Psychiatry 133:917–918, 1976

Strauss JS, Kokes RF, Klorman R, et al: Premorbid adjustment in schizophrenia: concepts, measures, and implications, part I: the concept of premorbid adjustment. Schizophr Bull 3:182–185, 1977

Straw RB: Meta-analysis of deinstitutionalization. Unpublished doctoral dissertation, Ann Arbor, MI, Northwestern University, 1982

Stroul BA: Crisis residential services in a community support system. Report to the NIMH Community Support Program. Rockville, MD, 1987

Sullivan H: Schizophrenia as a Human Process. New York, WW Norton, 1962

Szasz T: The Myth of Mental Illness: Foundations of a Theory of a Personal Conduct. New York, Hoeber-Harper, 1961

Taube C: General hospital inpatient psychiatric services 1967. Survey and Reports Section, Biometry Branch, Office of Program Planning and Evaluation, NIMH, Rockville, MD, 1969

Taube C: Length of stay of discharges from general hospital psychiatric inpatient units, United States 1970–1971 (Statistical Note 70). Biometry Branch, NIMH, Rockville, MD, 1973

Vaillant G: Prospective prediction of schizophrenic remission. Arch Gen Psychiatry 11:509–515, 1964

Venables P, O'Connor N: A short scale for rating paranoid schizophrenia. Journal of Mental Science 105:815–818, 1959

Wendt J, Mosher LR, Matthews S, et al: A comparison of two treatment environments for schizophrenia, in Psychiatric Milieu and the Therapeutic Process. Edited by Gunderson JG, Will OA Jr, Mosher LR. New York, Jason Aronson, 1983, pp 17–33

The Pilot Project "Soteria Berne": Clinical Experiences and Results

Editor's Note

Soteria Berne, a Swiss therapeutic household for the treatment of patients with recent-onset schizophrenia, borrows many ideas from the Soteria Project described in the previous chapter. Like the California-based Soteria, the household in Berne aims to manage the illness in a small supportive environment, using neuroleptic medication in low doses and only in unusual circumstances. As in the earlier Soteria Project, the outcome of treatment in this domestic setting, with very restricted use of antipsychotic medication, is equivalent to that in a standard hospital or with outpatient care. An important lesson of both the Swiss and American Soteria Projects is that remission often occurs in patients with early schizophrenia without the use of neuroleptic medication if patients are managed in a supportive and human-scale environment.

The Pilot Project "Soteria Berne": Clinical Experiences and Results

Luc Ciompi, M.D.
Hans-Peter Dauwalder, Ph.D.
Christian Maier, M.D.
Elisabeth Aebi, lic. phil.
Karl Trütsch, M.D.
Zeno Kupper, Ph.D.
Charlotte Rutishauser, lic. phil.

*W*e still do not know enough about the etiology and pathogenesis of schizophrenia, and the therapeutic methods generated by our definition are not satisfactory. Therefore, innovative approaches to treating schizophrenic patients, even if they only promise some partial progress, warrant consideration. The purpose of the pilot project "Soteria Berne" is to assess the effectiveness of an open residential program that has been providing mainly psychotherapy, sociotherapy, and milieu therapy instead of standard pharmacotherapy to about 60 patients with acute schizophrenia for more than 6 years.

The project is based on three underlying concepts: First, a multi-conditional understanding of schizophrenia, generated by Ciompi's investigations (1987, 1988a, 1991) of the long-term course of illness and by his concept of "affect logic," according to which affects (or emotions) organize and integrate cognitions with which they are comprehensively linked; second, experiences reported by American authors

This description of the initial results of the program was first published in "The Pilot Project 'Soteria Berne': Clinical Experiences and Results." British Journal of Psychiatry 161(suppl 18):145–153, 1992. It is reproduced here with permission.

in the 1970s in the first Soteria House near San Francisco; and third, a number of other psychotherapeutic, sociotherapeutic, and pharmacological strategies that have been developed by other investigators.

The three-phase multiconditional evolutionary model of schizophrenia that has been described elsewhere (Ciompi 1983, 1987, 1988b) is based on a modified version of the vulnerability theory formulated by Zubin and Spring (1977), Nuechterlein and Dawson (1984), and others. Schizophrenic patients are defined as highly sensitive individuals with impaired information-processing capacities, which reduces their ability to cope with critical life events such as leaving home, first sexual experiences, choosing a job or a spouse, pregnancy and childbirth, and major changes in residence or life circumstances. Under unfavorable conditions, escalating emotional tensions between the patient and the environment reach a critical point of instability, characterized by the appearance of acute psychotic symptoms. Psychotic decompensation can be defined as a severe developmental crisis, bearing the risk of total failure, while providing a chance to grow and change.

This model has the following therapeutic implications: patients with this type of crisis need continual psychotherapeutic help and emotional support. Their difficulties in information processing should be alleviated in a calm, relaxing, and stimulus-reducing therapeutic setting, where a stable team ensures continuity and provides patients and their families with clear and reliable information about the illness. However, repeated change in therapeutic setting and therapist; emotional or intellectual overstimulation (Wing and Brown 1970); high "expressed emotion" in the family (see Leff et al. 1982); and confusing and contradictory information about the therapeutic situation, the purpose of therapy, and the methods employed should be avoided as much as possible. Therefore, the confusing and violent atmosphere endemic in the large admission wards of psychiatric hospitals, where a majority of acutely psychotic patients are still being treated, is particularly unsatisfactory. Small treatment facilities offering a sheltered and supportive environment may be more effective in treating schizophrenic patients than such traditional settings.

Background

The San Francisco Soteria House project, conceived by Mosher and Menn in the 1970s and investigated by a U.S. National Institute of

Mental Health study (see Chapter 7), has produced positive results (Matthews et al. 1979; Mosher and Menn 1978; Mosher et al. 1975, 1990; Wilson 1982)—the need for neuroleptic treatment was dramatically reduced. The outcome of treatment was predominantly positive for about 200 acute schizophrenic patients maintained on low-dose or no neuroleptic medication. After 6 weeks, no significant differences in the level of psychopathology could be found between 28 index patients treated without drugs and 11 control patients receiving a daily average dose of 700 mg of chlorpromazine equivalents (Mosher et al. 1990); after 2 years, no significant differences were reported in relapse rates or psychopathology. However, the index patients had a better level of social adjustment, were less distressed by their illness, were using significantly lower total doses of neuroleptic drugs, and incurred lower treatment costs. These findings, which are interesting in connection with the problem of both short-term and long-term side effects of neuroleptic drugs, have to date not been systematically analyzed or replicated.

The project discussed here borrowed certain therapeutic and administrative tools, such as the "soft room" and nurses' timetables (see "Method" below), from the initial Soteria experiment. The same name (a rough translation from the Greek, meaning safety, security, salvation) was used, despite the fact that Soteria Berne differs from Mosher's approach in various ways; it is based on a medical model integrating psychosocial and biological factors, it is under medical supervision, and it incorporates the following therapeutic strategies: 1) the "educational approach" and family treatment strategy (Anderson 1983; Hubschmid 1985; Leff et al. 1982), intended to establish close collaboration between family, significant others, and health care professionals; 2) long-term aftercare and relapse prevention (Dauwalder 1988); 3) inducing positive expectations (Ciompi et al. 1979) by providing everyone involved in the therapy process with clear and updated information about the illness, its treatment, the long-term risk of relapse, and the chance of recovery, according to follow-up studies that have demonstrated that long-term outcome is substantially more favorable and heterogeneous than hitherto believed (Bleuler 1978; Ciompi and Müller 1976; Huber et al. 1979); and 4) administration of low-dose and targeted medication as viable alternatives to drug-free strategies (Carpenter et al. 1977, 1987, 1990; Chiles et al. 1989; Herz et al. 1982; Kane and Lieberman 1987; Kane et al. 1983).

The combination of these strategies generated the following eight therapeutic fundamentals of Soteria Berne:

1. Continuous human and psychotherapeutic support in a therapeutic setting that is as normal as possible—small, relaxing, harmonious, and nonstimulating
2. Stable and supportive interpersonal bonds with a few carefully selected persons during the psychotic crisis
3. A stable team of staff members who apply a consistent concept of therapy beginning with the acute phase of treatment up to social and vocational rehabilitation
4. Continuous close collaboration with relatives and significant others
5. The same information about illness, prognosis, and treatment given to patients, relatives, and care providers
6. Joint negotiation of concrete goals and priorities about projected living and job arrangements, and establishment of realistic and cautious prospects for the future
7. Use of neuroleptic drugs only in cases of acute danger to oneself or to others, if there are no signs of improvement within 3–4 weeks, or to prevent an impending relapse in the aftercare phase
8. Systematic aftercare and relapse prevention over a period of at least 2 years, based on a combined effort by the patient, family members, and care providers to recognize the individual's characteristic prodromal symptoms and the situations that tend to overtax his or her coping resources, and potential modes of dealing with difficult situations

Method

Soteria Berne opened on May 1, 1984, in a 12-room house with a garden in the middle of Berne. The house can accommodate a maximum of six to eight patients and two nurses. Patients admitted had to meet the following criteria:

- Age 17–35 years
- A recent onset of a schizophrenic or schizophreniform psychosis defined according to DSM-III-R (American Psychiatric Association 1987) criteria not more than 1 year before admission

- At least two of the following six symptoms within the previous 4 weeks: delusions, hallucinations, thought disorders, catatonia, schizophrenic disorders of affect, and severely deviant social behavior

The exclusion criteria consisted of dependency on drugs or alcohol and total lack of compliance with treatment.

Referral to Soteria is usually made by the local emergency service, but patients are also sometimes referred by local psychiatric hospitals or private professionals. Random admission is attempted by accepting patients who fulfill the above-mentioned criteria whenever a bed is available. However, some bias is created by the fact that severely agitated acute patients are quite often directly referred to nearby psychiatric hospitals without passing through the emergency service, and compulsory treatment is generally not possible in the open Soteria setting. Furthermore, some patients with longer-lasting illnesses, chronic course, and severe negative symptoms have been admitted under different circumstances. Therefore, the index population may have contained patients who were somewhat easier to treat, but also with less favorable outcome prospects than a typical population of acute patients with a shorter duration of illness and no severe negative symptoms.

The therapeutic team consists of a part-time medical director, five psychiatric nurses, and four paraprofessionals selected according to their motivation, life experience, and ability to show empathy and interpersonal involvement with schizophrenic patients. Two staff members always work in overlapping 48-hour shifts followed by several days off. The team has weekly half-day meetings to review cases. Once every 2 weeks an experienced psychotherapist supervises the team.

Treatment is divided into four phases; each patient is assigned a health care professional who stays constantly with him or her during the initial and most acute phase. Care begins in the "soft room," a large and pleasant room on the ground floor. This room has only cushions and mattresses, to prevent danger or overstimulation. The main purpose of this phase is to calm the patient and to reduce anxiety and tension by providing constant human support and guidance or by implementing relaxation techniques such as massage, holding hands, short walks, or other physical activities. Next is the *activating phase,* characterized by gradually getting the patient back into touch with reality—first by negotiating simple household and gardening chores within the sheltered environment of the therapeutic setting, and later by going shopping and for walks near the house. The *third phase* focuses on gradual social and vocational rehabilitation by expanding the patient's social network and helping him or her to make the transition from hospital to independent living by providing part-time employment or placement in a sheltered workshop. The *fourth phase,* which lasts for at least 2 years after discharge, focuses on prevention of relapse and psychosocial stabilization. It is carried out by a mobile community-based social-psychiatric team or by private psychiatrists.

Psychosocial therapy focuses on the patient's basic life problems and on treating the psychosis as an integral part of the patient's life. At the beginning, each patient is offered ongoing support and guidance as required, by two health care providers who are specifically assigned to do this. Eventually, individual or family therapy might be offered, according to the circumstances. Relatives and significant others are systematically involved in the therapy process; they are informed about the illness whenever an appropriate situation arises, and information is also disseminated in problem-centered workshops that take place every 6 weeks. Psychoanalytical and systemic family therapeutic approaches continually influence psychosocial interventions—for example, in efforts to strengthen personal identity, to clarify intrafamilial responsibilities, to reinforce interpersonal and generational boundaries, or to negotiate concrete priorities and objectives, such as housing or vocational arrangements.

Results

The following results are available: clinical observations, some data concerning the immediate outcome on discharge of 60 patients treated at Soteria between May 1, 1984, and April 30, 1990, and outcome comparisons over a 2-year period between the first 14 index and control patients. More detailed information, including methods, is found elsewhere in a German-language publication (Ciompi et al. 1991).

At the reference date of April 30, 1990, 56 of 60 patients treated (36 women and 24 men ages 17.7–36.5 years, mean 23.8 years, SD 3.5 years) had been discharged. Of these, 39 met DSM-III-R criteria for schizophrenia and 14 for schizophreniform psychosis (three diagnoses were uncertain). The duration of illness varied widely, averaging 1.37 years (SD 2.52); duration of treatment at Soteria varied between 3 and

765 days (mean 153.8 days, SD 169.9 days). The great majority of patients stayed at Soteria for an average of 1 to 4 months (Figure 8–1).

On the whole, the first three phases of the treatment approach may be considered quite successful. Patients incurred serious harm to themselves or to others in only three incidents in 6 years. Several patients who remained drug-free for a period ranging from several weeks to a number of months had less severe psychotic symptoms, although the time spans for this effect to occur were usually longer than those reported by Mosher and colleagues (1975; Mosher and Menn 1978). This was one of the reasons for the increased implementation of targeted or low-dose neuroleptic medication strategies as time passed. However, relapse prevention often proved to be more difficult than expected during the aftercare phase of the program. This was mainly because many patients and their relatives refused to acknowledge either the patient's special vulnerability or the necessity of guidance and care, even though they had been informed about the nature of the illness. Medication was, therefore, administered on an as-needed basis during this phase of treatment.

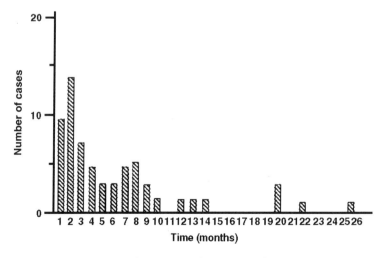

Figure 8–1. Duration of treatment of patients at Soteria Berne.

Five of the 56 patients were discharged within 10 days and were therefore not included in the statistical analysis. Twenty of the 51 remaining patients received no neuroleptic treatment at Soteria, and 31 received neuroleptic drugs for approximately two-thirds of their stay, in average daily doses of 172.5 mg of chlorpromazine equivalents (calculated according to Haase 1982) or 94.2 mg/day of total treatment. This corresponds to approximately one-third of the usual European doses, and about one-fifth to one-tenth of the usual American doses. Psychopathology on release, housing situation and occupational situation after release, and a global outcome rating are shown in Table 8–1.

In 31 (61%) out of 51 patients, the immediate global outcome was classified as "good," or "fairly good," and in 18 (35.3%) as "rather poor" or "poor," suggesting that the program was successful in a major subgroup, but unsuccessful in a minor subgroup of psychotic patients. Immediate outcome is shown in Figure 8–2.

A number of significant differences were found between "responders" and "nonresponders" (Table 8–2): for certain aspects of outcome, there were better results in women than in men, in patients with a shorter duration of illness, and in schizophreniform psychoses versus schizophrenia defined according to DSM-III-R criteria. Surprisingly, patients who received no or very low dosage medication demonstrated significantly better results. Additional statistical comparisons between "extreme" subgroups (category 1 versus category 4) and a number of nonsignificant trends point in the same direction.

Comparisons were made of the 2-year outcomes between the first 14 index patients and an equal number of matched control patients from four different institutions (the milieu therapy–oriented private psychiatric hospital Schlössli in Oetwil, Switzerland; a modern psychiatric ward at Lucerne General Hospital in Switzerland; the traditional state psychiatric hospital in St. Urban, Lucerne, in Switzerland; and the state psychiatric hospital Philips-Hospital near Riedstadt in Germany). The Ward Atmosphere Scale (Henrich et al. 1979; Moos 1974) significantly differentiated Soteria from the four control institutions with respect to therapeutic atmosphere (Figure 8–3).

Matched-pair comparisons were made by matching index and control patients with respect to their age, sex, and the two most relevant predictors, premorbid social adjustment and prevailing positive or negative symptoms. The results of this comparison are summarized in

Figure 8–4; no significant differences were found for seven out of a total of nine outcome and progression variables. The variables included

1. Psychopathology measured by the Brief Psychiatric Rating Scale (BPRS) (Overall and Gorham 1962)
2. Housing situation
3. Job situation
4. Global outcome combining variables 1–3

Table 8–1. Measures of outcome for patients

Measure	No. of cases
Psychopathology	
Category	
1: no psychotic symptoms (full remission)	21
2: minimal residuals	12
3: medium residuals	7
4: no improvement, or impairment	4
5: uncertain	7
Housing situation	
Category	
1: normal housing situation (alone or with colleagues)	19
2: with parents	14
3: sheltered community or halfway home	6
4: psychiatric hospital	9
5: uncertain	3
Occupational situation	
Category	
1: normal work or school	20
2: part-time work	5
3: sheltered workshop or rehabilitation center	5
4: unoccupied	19
5: uncertain	2
Global outcome rating	
1. good (category 1 or 2 in all three ratings)	19
2. rather good (category 1 or 2 in two of three ratings)	12
3. rather poor (category 3 or 4 in two of three ratings)	9
4. poor (category 3 or 4 in three ratings)	9
5. uncertain (category "uncertain" in two or three ratings)	2

5. Global autonomy score—score comprised of 1) legal responsibility, 2) living along or with one's family, 3) job and financial situation, 4) recreational activities, and 5) social contacts (see Hubschmid and Aebi 1986)
6. Relapse rate
7. Average treatment costs

In both groups, 10 out of 14 patients (71.4%) had relapses over 2 years; 9 index patients and 7 control patients had to be readmitted as day or inpatients. The only significant differences were for mean daily dose ($P < .01$) and total dose ($P < .05$).

Seven out of 14 index patients and all 14 control patients received neuroleptic treatment during the initial inpatient treatment phase. During aftercare, 8 out of 14 index patients and 12 out of 14 control patients were treated with neuroleptics. Four index patients did not receive neuroleptics either during the initial treatment phase or during aftercare; all four patients had symptoms diagnosed as schizophreniform psychoses and had a good outcome. Index patients received significantly smaller daily and cumulative neuroleptic doses than control patients. During the inpatient phase, the respective differences amounted to more than 1:30 (81 mg versus 2,615 mg average daily dose) and more than 1:7 (14.694 mg versus 105.198 mg average total dose), whereas no significant differences were found during aftercare (99 mg versus 103 mg average daily dose, and 68.968 mg versus 67.713 mg average total dose, respectively) (Figure 8–4). During the total 2-year period of observation, the difference in average total doses between index and control patients was about 1:2 (83.662 mg versus 172.911 mg).

Correlations found between possible predictors and housing situation, job situation, psychopathology, and combined global outcome are shown in Table 8–3.

Better outcomes (partly for both index patients and control patients, and partly only for the one or the other) were statistically correlated with being female, above-average age, higher professional training, better premorbid social functioning, higher premorbid autonomy, shorter duration of illness and of previous treatment, and absence of previous psychotic episodes. In terms of medication, outcomes were statistically better for patients who did not receive neuroleptics during aftercare, or who received them for a shorter-than-average duration and at higher-than-average doses during the treatment phase, but at lower-than-average doses during aftercare. Furthermore, index patients who received lower-than-average total doses during the treatment phase had statistically better outcomes.

On the whole, almost all correlations concerning general and social predictors were in the direction expected according to the literature (e.g., Hubschmid and Ciompi 1990). However, the correlations contradicted expectations concerning the absence of the predictive power of diagnostic subgroups and the generally more favorable aspects of outcome for patients who were maintained on targeted low-dose or nonneuroleptic medication strategies.

Discussion

More than 6 years of experience with a significantly sized group of schizophrenic patients shows that the innovative therapeutic approach implemented in Soteria Berne is applicable to clinical practice and, in terms of immediate outcome, has been successful in about two-thirds of cases. It is particularly interesting that for certain patients, a remission of symptoms can occur without neuroleptic medication, and that

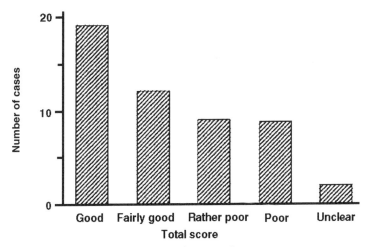

Figure 8–2.   Immediate outcomes for 51 patients.

drug-free or low-dose medication strategies have been correlated with better outcomes in several respects. The results of the 2-year prospective study on the first 14 index patients and matched control subjects are also surprising insofar as they show no significant differences

Table 8–2.   Correlations between possible predictors and immediate outcomes

	Housing (*n* = 48)	Work (*n* = 49)	Psychopathology (*n* = 44)	Total score (*n* = 49)
Sex (men/women)	NS	NS	NS	-.349*
Age (< 24 years/ > 24 years)	NS	NS	NS	NS
Duration of illness (< 1 year/ > 1 year)	.337*	NS	NS	NS
Diagnosis (schizophrenia/ schizophreniform psychosis)	NS	NS	-.321*	NS
Duration of treatment (< 6 months/ > 6 months)	NS	NS	NS	NS
Neuroleptic medication (no/yes)	NS	.323*	NS	.317*
Duration of medication (< mean/ > mean)	NS	NS	NS	NS
Mean dose (< 172 mg/ > 172 mg)	NS	NS	NS	NS
Total dose (< mean/ > mean)	NS	NS	NS	NS

Note.   NS = not significant.
*$P < .05$.

between standard treatment and the Soteria approach with respect to psychopathology, housing arrangements, job situation, combined global outcome, social autonomy, and relapse rate, despite much smaller daily and total doses of neuroleptic medication. This confirms findings by Mosher et al. (1975, 1990) and by Mosher and Menn (1978). On the other hand, treatment costs were significantly higher for the Soteria patients.

It appears that in a special therapeutic setting that offers adequate and continual emotional support, long-term comparable outcomes can be achieved despite a substantial reduction in the cumulative use of

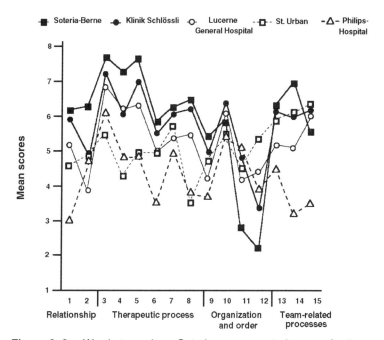

Figure 8–3. Ward atmosphere Soteria versus control groups for the following factors: 1) involvement, 2) spontaneity, 3) autonomy, 4) practical orientation, 5) orientation to the future, 6) therapists as models, 7) reinforcement, 8) scope of program, 9) transparency of concepts, 10) transparency of program, 11) control by staff, 12) order and organization, 13) team coherence, 14) team hierarchy, and 15) team information flow.

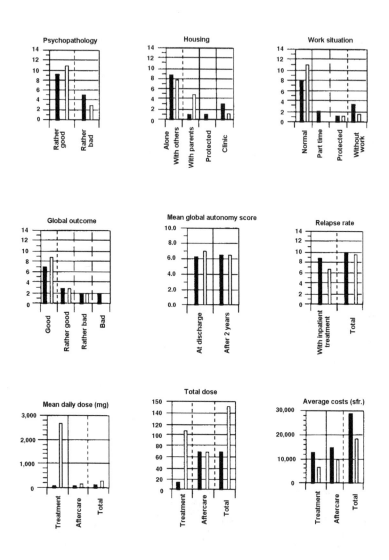

Figure 8–4. Comparison of index (■) and control (❑) patients after 2 years.

Table 8–3. Soteria Berne: Correlations between possible predictors and 2-year outcome

	Housing	Work	Psychopathology	Total score
Sex (men/women)	−0.51*[a]	0.38*[b]	NS	NS
Age (< 24 years/> 24 years)	NS	NS	NS	−0.37*
Diagnosis (schizophrenia/schizophreniform psychosis)	NS	NS	NS	NS
Professional formation (low/high)	NS	NS	−0.56*[b]	NS
Premorbid social functioning (low/high)	−0.57*[b]	NS	NS	NS
Psychosocial autonomy (low/high)	−0.53*[b]	NS	NS	NS
Outbreak of illness (< 6 months/> 6 months)	0.61**[c]	NS	NS	NS
Previous treatment (< 6 months/> 6 months)	0.55*[c]	NS	NS	NS
Previous psychotic episodes (no/yes)	0.54*[c]	NS	NS	NS
Neuroleptic medication				
Treatment: (no/yes)	NS	NS	NS	NS
Aftercare: (no/yes)	0.51**[a]	NS	0.64*[c]	0.58*
Duration of medication				
Treatment: (</> 61 days)	0.56**[a]	0.47*[a]	NS	0.49*[a]
Aftercare: (</> 284 days)	NS	NS	NS	NS
Mean dose				
Treatment: (</> 258 mg)	NS	0.73*[c]	NS	NS
Aftercare: (</> 292 mg)	1.00*[b]	0.67*[b]	NS	0.67*[b]
Total dose				
Treatment: (</> 15 g)	1.00***[c]	NS	0.73*[c]	0.73*[c]
Aftercare: (</> 69 g)	NS	NS	NS	NS

Note. NS = not significant.
[a]All patients (*n* = 28). [b]Control patients (*n* = 14). [c]Index patients (*n* = 14).
* *P* < .05. ** *P* < .01. *** *P* < .001.

medication; some drug-free patients have positive outcomes after 2 years of study. This finding is particularly interesting with regard to tardive dyskinesia, which has some relationship to the cumulative neuroleptics administered (Carpenter et al. 1990). The findings reported are compatible with the hypothesis of central organizing and integrating functions of the affects (Ciompi 1991) and partially validate the underlying psychosociobiological understanding of schizophrenia derived from the concept of "affect logic" (Ciompi 1988a, 1988b). A unilaterally biological concept of schizophrenia would hardly suffice to explain them.

These findings, however, should be interpreted with great caution. Statistical correlations in favor of patients who received no or low-dose neuroleptic medication do not provide evidence for the hypothesis that drug-free treatment is superior to conventional neuroleptic medication strategies, because only more difficult patients were given neuroleptics or higher doses of them. Furthermore, the number of matched-pair comparisons over 2 years was small, and the influence of important mediating variables such as duration and dosage of medication, environmental influences, and spontaneous remission rates has not yet been sufficiently investigated.

The near-identical relapse rates for both medication strategies can be explained by the fact that both groups were maintained on almost identical total-dose levels during aftercare. Therefore, slightly higher rates of readmission among index patients cannot be related to differences in drug prophylaxis. Soteria patients might, however, be less reluctant to return to the treatment facility than patients treated in traditional hospitals.

Higher treatment costs in Soteria probably have less to do with the low- or no-medication strategies adopted than with the prolongation of treatment, caused by the inclusion of phase 3 (rehabilitation) in the treatment process. Furthermore, higher initial costs are to be expected in a pilot project. It is certainly possible to reduce costs by referring patients to less expensive rehabilitation facilities; this has already been initiated. However, in the face of the immeasurable human and economic costs of the unsolved problem of schizophrenia, financial reasons alone should certainly not hinder the search for improved therapeutic methods.

Although it appears that under emotionally favorable conditions, a low- or no-medication strategy, combined with psychotherapy and sociotherapy, is a feasible and effective alternative to conventional treatment for schizophrenic patients, the question of how to differentiate "responders" from "nonresponders" has not yet been clarified. Some findings (better results for schizophreniform psychoses, women, and premorbidly more autonomous first-episode cases with short duration of illness and no previous treatment elsewhere) support the assumption that a drug-free treatment condition, focusing on milieu therapy and psychotherapy, may be more suitable for new patients with less severe disorders. Moreover, the fact that the last three predictors of favorable outcome are valid only for index patients and not for control patients (see Table 8–2) suggests that this therapeutic approach might be suitable mainly for patients who did not have the opportunity to learn the typical roles and behavioral patterns characteristic of psychiatric inpatients.

Finally, on the subjective level of experience, most patients and relatives found treatment at Soteria to be less upsetting and less stigmatizing than traditional methods. Apparently, Soteria patients could more easily integrate their psychosis into their lives and personal development than could patients being treated in customary psychiatric facilities.

Overall, the findings reported provide some hope of improving methods of treatment for at least one major subgroup of psychotic patients by using the Soteria approach.

References

American Psychiatric Association: Diagnostic and Statistical Manual of Mental Disorders, 3rd Edition, Revised. Washington, DC, American Psychiatric Association, 1987

Anderson C: A psychoeducational model of family treatment for schizophrenia, in Psychosocial Intervention in Schizophrenia. Edited by Stierlin H, Wynne LC, Wirshing M. Berlin, Springer, 1983, pp 227–234

Bleuler M: The Schizophrenic Disorders: Long-Term Patient and Family Studies. New Haven, CT, Yale University Press, 1978

Carpenter WT, McGlashan TH, Strauss JS: The treatment of acute schizophrenia without drugs: an investigation of some current assumptions. Am J Psychiatry 134:14–20, 1977

Carpenter WT, Heinrichs DW, Hanlon TE: A comparative trial of pharmacologic strategies in schizophrenia. Am J Psychiatry 144:1466–1470, 1987

Carpenter WT, Heinrichs DW, Hanlon TE, et al: Continuous versus targeted medication in schizophrenic outpatients: outcome results. Am J Psychiatry 147:1138–1148, 1990

Chiles JA, Sterchi D, Hyde T, et al: Intermittent medication for schizophrenic outpatients: who is eligible? Schizophr Bull 15:117–120, 1989

Ciompi L: How to improve the treatment of schizophrenics: a multicausal illness concept and its therapeutic consequences, in Psychosocial Intervention in Schizophrenia. Edited by Stierlin H, Wynne LC, Wirsching M. Berlin, Springer, 1983, pp 53–63

Ciompi L: Toward a coherent multidimensional understanding and therapy of schizophrenia: converging new concepts, in Psychosocial Treatment. Edited by Strauss JS, Böker W, Brenner HD. Toronto, Huber, 1987, pp 43–62

Ciompi L: The Psyche and Schizophrenia: The Bond Between Affect and Logic. Cambridge, MA, Harvard University Press, 1988a

Ciompi L: Learning from outcome studies: toward a comprehensive biological-psychosocial understanding of schizophrenia. Schizophr Res 1:373–384, 1988b

Ciompi L: Affects as central organizing and integrating factors: a new psychosocial/biological model of the psyche. Br J Psychiatry 159:97–105, 1991

Ciompi L, Müller C: Lebensweg und Alter der Schizophrenen: Eine Katamnestische Langzeitstudie bis ins Alter. Berlin, Springer, 1976

Ciompi L, Dauwalder HP, Ague C: Ein Forschungsprogramm zur Rehabilitation psychisch Kranker, III: Längsschnittuntersuchungen zum Rehabilitationserfolg und zur Prognostik. Nervenarzt 50:366–378, 1979

Ciompi L, Dauwalder HP, Maier CH, et al: Das Pilotprojekt "Soteria Bern" zur Behandlung akut Schizophrener. Nervenartzt 62:428–435, 1991

Dauwalder HP: Psychische Gesundheit: Warum "präventives Verhalten" und nicht "Prävention"? erfahrungen aus der Sekundärprävention der Schizophrenie, in Lebensweltbezogene Prävention. Edited by Start W. Freiburg, Lambertus, 1988, pp 293–304

Haase HJ: Therapie mit Psychopharmaka und anderen seelisches Befinden beeinflussenden Medikamenten, 2nd Edition. Stuttgart, Schattauer, 1982

Henrich G, De Jong R, Mai N, et al: Aspekte des therapeutischen Klimas—Entwicklung eines Fragebogens. Z Klin Psychol Psychopathol Psychother 8:41–55, 1979

Herz MJ, Szymanski HV, Simon YC: Intermittent medication for stable schizophrenic outpatients: an alternative to maintenance medication. Am J Psychiatry 139:918–922, 1982

Huber G, Gross G, Schuettler R: Schizophrenie. Eine verlaufsund sozialpsychiatrische Langzeitstudie. Berlin, Springer, 1979

Hubschmid T: Von der Familientherapie zur Angehörigenarbeit oder vom therapeutischen zum präventiv-rehabilitativen Paradigma in der Schizophreniebenhandlung. Fortschr Neurol Psychiatr 53:117–122, 1985

Hubschmid T, Aebi E: Berufliche Wiedereingliederung von psychiatrischen Langzeitpatienten. Eine katamnestische Untersuchung. Soc Psychiatry 21:152–157, 1986

Hubschmid T, Ciompi L: Prädiktoren des Schizophrenieverlaufseine Literaturübersicht. Fortschr Neurol Psychiatr 58:359–366, 1990

Kane JM, Lieberman JA: Maintenance pharmacotherapy in schizophrenia, in Psychopharmacology: The Third Generation of Progress. Edited by Meltzer HY. New York, Raven, 1987, pp 1103–1109

Kane JM, Rifkin A, Woerner M, et al: Low-dose neuroleptic treatment of outpatient schizophrenics, I: preliminary results for relapse rates. Arch Gen Psychiatry 40:893–896, 1983

Leff JP, Kuipers L, Berkowitz R, et al: A controlled trial of social intervention in the families of schizophrenic patients. Br J Psychiatry 141:121–134, 1982

Matthews SM, Roper MT, Mosher LR, et al: A non-neuroleptic treatment for schizophrenia: analysis of the two-year postdischarge risk of relapse. Schizophr Bull 5:322–333, 1979

Moos R: Evaluating Treatment Environments: A Social Ecological Approach. New York, Wiley, 1974

Mosher LR, Menn AJ: Community residential treatment for schizophrenia: two-year follow-up data. Hosp Community Psychiatry 29:715–723, 1978

Mosher LR, Menn AJ, Matthews S: Evaluation of a homebased treatment for schizophrenics. Am J Orthopsychiatry 45:455–467, 1975

Mosher LR, Vallone R, Menn A: The treatment of acute psychosis without neuroleptics: new data from the Soteria Project. Paper presented at the annual meeting of the American Psychiatric Association, New York, May 1990

Nuechterlein JH, Dawson ME: A heuristic vulnerability/stress model of schizophrenic episodes. Schizophr Bull 10:300–312, 1984

Overall JE, Gorham DR: The Brief Psychiatric Rating Scale. Psychol Rep 10:799–812, 1962

Wilson HS: Deinstitutionalized Residential Care for the Mentally Disordered. The Soteria House Approach. New York, Grune & Stratton, 1982

Wing JK, Brown GW: Institutionalism and Schizophrenia. London, Cambridge University Press, 1970

Zubin J, Spring B: Vulnerability—a new view on schizophrenia. J Abnorm Psychol 86:103–126, 1977

Burch House, Inc., Bethlehem, New Hampshire: History and Description

Editor's Note

Burch House is an independent treatment household in New Hampshire. Like the Soteria Project, it traces its origins back to Kingsley Hall in London and the work of R. D. Laing and his associates. The household is a therapeutic community with a family-style atmosphere; as in a family home, there is no strict schedule or prescribed daily routine, and residents may come and go freely. The household accepts people with diverse emotional problems, and some stay for a period of years. To a greater extent, perhaps, than any of the programs described so far in this book, the people at Burch House believe that psychosis is a transitional state that may lead to positive life change for the person experiencing it. On many occasions, the household has undertaken the care of severely disturbed psychotic people without recourse to neuroleptic medication, relying instead on the expectation that the homelike surroundings will have a healing effect.

Chapter 9

Burch House, Inc., Bethlehem, New Hampshire: History and Description

David B. Goldblatt, M.A.

*B*urch House is an alternative to psychiatric hospitalization for people who want to take responsibility for their own healing process and participate in a community where others help them change to make the most of their life. It is a 19-room home on 14 acres of land in Bethlehem, New Hampshire (Figure 9–1). Up to eight patients and four staff-members-in-training live together. They share the responsibilities of maintaining their home and attending to each other. It is a safe and supportive environment for patients to live through the healing process.

The house has 12 bedrooms and several large common rooms for unlimited activities, such as meetings, yoga, meditation, relaxation, and listening to or making music. A large, well-equipped kitchen has its own fireplace and a table that comfortably seats 16 people. It has a warm and cozy atmosphere that is very welcoming, relaxing, and calming. Most people who visit Burch House comment about how warm and comfortable it seems and how it exudes a feeling of safety.

Several of the common rooms have either a wood stove or a fireplace, which adds to the warm atmosphere. A laundry room is available for patients to wash and dry their clothes. Regular, nonpay telephones are easily accessible, although people are expected to pay for their long-distance calls. Each resident has a private bedroom that can be decorated as wished. We respect an individual's privacy and do not intrude into someone's personal space unless a serious emergency exists.

The Patients

The patients come from various backgrounds, and they present with a wide spectrum of diagnostic problems. They are referred by professionals, family, or friends or are self-referred. We do not discriminate against anyone who wants to come to Burch House, unless they are actively suicidal, violent toward others, or under the influence of alcohol or narcotic drugs. Potential residents addicted to alcohol or drugs must be free of them for at least 6 months before coming to Burch House. Burch House is a transitional facility, not a permanent residence.

Staffing

The staff comprises two full-time members who live outside the house, four interns who live in the house, and a part-time staff member whose primary role is fund-raising. The full-time or senior staff do some administrative work and spend time in the milieu and in one-on-one sessions with patients. These staff members may or may not have had

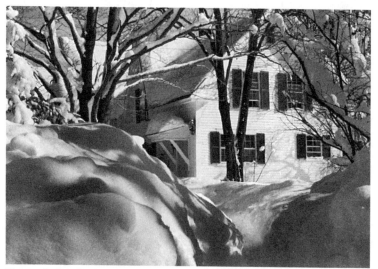

Figure 9–1. Burch House, Bethlehem, New Hampshire.

formal training prior to their employment at Burch House; this has varied over the years—people have had graduate degrees, undergraduate degrees, or no degree at all. The interns are trained by the senior staff or sometimes by outside sources and by the experience of living and working at Burch House. Senior staff positions are often filled by people who were interns. There has not been much turnover among the senior staff: they tend to stay with us a long time.

Background

Burch House was conceived by Catherine (Katy) Burch Symmes and me around 1970. We were both faculty members at Franconia College, a small, innovative, liberal arts college. We had had many experiences with students in serious emotional trouble and found that sending these people to a hospital rarely improved their situation. Both Katy and I occasionally brought students who were having a hard time into our own homes for short periods of time. I believe that we helped dozens of students by giving them a safe haven for a short period of time.

During my years of teaching college and earlier in graduate school, I had developed a fascination with the work of R. D. Laing and the establishment of Kingsley Hall in London. Kingsley Hall, started by the psychiatrists R. D. Laing and Aaron Esterson, was a British experimental psychiatric alternative in which patients and therapists lived together and virtually anything was permitted (Barnes and Berke 1972).

In London, I spent 4 years training with R. D. Laing and the Philadelphia Association and working in the therapeutic communities they had established (Cooper 1989). This is where the sense of what our community was going to be began to crystallize. The essential principle on which Burch House was founded was that individuals would be provided with a sanctuary in which they could "get back on their feet" without being given a particular diagnosis or method of treatment. We wanted to see if a supportive relationship and a safe environment were enough to heal patients with emotional illness.

Early in my training with the Philadelphia Association I was brought into one of the communities to "be with" a woman who had become psychotic. "Being with" someone refers to one of the most important aspects of this work. Some people grasp the concept immediately, whereas others struggle for years trying to learn how to be with someone while not interfering with his or her process.

I was faced with the situation of a naked woman on the floor who was digging her fingers into her anus to obtain small globs of feces that she was smearing on her hair and face. I sat with her for a while without knowing what was going to happen next or what to do. I was not frightened for either her or me. Although she was engaged in an activity that made no sense to me, I assumed that it made some sense to her. After a short period of time, I asked her if she would let me help her take a bath. To my surprise, she agreed and even seemed to welcome the attention and caring.

I described this situation to illustrate how people can be deeply disturbed or engage in bizarre behavior, and with simple human contact, return to a stable state. If people go through a crisis with the support of empathic, caring, and compassionate fellow human beings, then those people will develop the strength necessary to deal with the difficulties, agonies, and fears of life. It may require a person to stay up all night with someone in crisis rather than to prescribe a drug to calm his or her nerves, even if the patient is dealing with his or her most dreaded demons. In many situations, this approach is not possible, but, in most instances, people in crisis should be given the opportunity to work in this way if they wish.

For about 2 weeks, this woman remained in a psychotic state, often staying up all night, frequently speaking what seemed to be nonsense, often struggling with the people who stayed with her, and, occasionally, trying to run out of the house. Gradually, she began to communicate with those people taking turns being with her, and, gradually, she began to "clear" from her psychosis.

In London, I had seen many people who successfully experienced the therapeutic community. It gave them the space and time to be who they were, even if it meant being lost and admitting it for the first time, and it permitted them to go through a healing process in a safe environment. I became excited to see if we could reproduce these results in the United States. Aside from Loren Mosher's and Alma Menn's work with Soteria (Mosher and Menn 1978) and John Perry's work with Diabasis, I had not heard of other alternatives in North America. I now know of some that are more recent and of many communities that are not alternatives to the mainstream.

Essentially, we wanted a safe environment where people could go through whatever process they needed or wanted. There seems to be a natural human tendency to help or to "fix" someone who appears to be in trouble. I have realized that because someone is lost or says they are lost does not translate into "find me" or "help me." We wanted to create a safe environment, not a treatment facility. I will try to describe how we did this and some of what we learned, but I forewarn you that a lot of our original idealism and naivety has changed. In retrospect, it was easy to be naive because there was virtually no precedent for what we were attempting to demonstrate and accomplish.

Program Description

Burch House is located about a 30-minute walk from the center of a small New England town, Littleton, New Hampshire, with an overall population of about 7,500. It is a relatively peaceful town where there is seldom any trouble or reason to feel unsafe. You can take a walk at any time of the day or night. The winter can be cold and relatively long, but it can also be very beautiful. There are four distinct seasons, each with its own beauty. The area is the White Mountains of New Hampshire, and a variety of outdoor activities are available.

Burch House maintains a large vegetable garden and smaller flower and herb gardens around the house. The people who live and work at Burch House do all the cleaning and maintaining of the inside and outside of the house. The work schedule we have is minimal and flexible to adjust for personal needs; it is not strict and there is no specific daily routine. People have a tremendous amount of free time to design their own day, week, or month. Everyone is expected to be involved and to be part of the community.

Burch House has many kinds of activities, and people are involved in various ways. The extent of involvement may vary from person to person or from one time period to another. Residents are free to come and go from Burch House any time. However, we do expect that people who live at Burch House participate in the house in a variety of ways—to help with chores, to be there for their own therapy in some form, and to be involved in the milieu and not seclude themselves for extensive periods. At a house meeting held once a week, everyone signs up for either an indoor chore, such as cleaning a public area or bathroom in the house, or an outdoor chore, such as mowing the lawn, bringing in firewood, or working in the garden. In addition, we sign up for cooking one evening meal each week and cleaning the kitchen 1 day each week. The cooking involves some planning because one must go shopping or prepare a shopping list.

During the week, three other community meetings are held in addition to the house meeting. These meetings can be used for any purpose that those involved want. This means possibly discussing personal issues, house issues, or even philosophy. The important thing is that people attend. Patients can also meet with a therapist outside of the house or with one or two staff members together. We encourage family meetings periodically if this is appropriate.

The fact that we are a community is taken seriously, and everyone is expected to be part of that community, or Burch House is not appropriate for them. This approach comes from years of experience showing us that certain situations actually work against the well-being and well-functioning of Burch House as a therapeutic community. There is still latitude and space for individuals to be themselves, however, and to go through what they may need to in their own time and way, provided that way does not seriously threaten or damage anyone else's or the community's well-being.

This may have a ring of imposed schedules or regulations from some authority, but this is not so. Virtually all decisions are community decisions, which means patients and staff decide together. There are very few rules, except those that involve being mindful and respectful of another's space and well-being.

Treatment

The issue of medication use at Burch House is between a patient and her or his doctor. Medications have always been a touchy issue, and there has been a lot of misconception and even rumor about our position on this subject.

Essentially, we do not support the misuse and excessive use of medication for any reason. There are no medical staff at Burch House, so we cannot prescribe medications or say how they are to be used. We do have many years of experience working with individuals in distress or in a variety of disturbed and disturbing states and have seen many instances of medications being used to treat emotional distress. We do not believe that emotional distress has a biological cause, except in some circumstances, so medications are seen as the exception rather than the rule for the individual in distress.

We do believe that in some instances, medications can be helpful for either short or long periods of time, and that special circumstances require the use of medications for very long or even lifelong duration; this may have beneficial effects on an individual's well-being and peace of mind.

"Peace of mind" is not always the best solution, however, because sometimes suffering or being troubled is a path to healing. But we acknowledge that sometimes enough is enough. Those decisions are mutual, and we never tell someone how to act at Burch House unless the situation is life threatening or so disturbing to others at the house that it cannot be tolerated. Again, I absolutely acknowledge that medication can be a valuable tool during a difficult period, particularly when someone is on their own and does not have a support network.

The use of medication by someone who has had a major emotional distress for many years is very different from the use by someone who has recently either broken down or who has never taken medications. It has been our experience that when someone has never used medication and/or has only recently had emotional problems, that they are more likely to become emotionally balanced without medication than someone who has used medications for years who tries to become balanced without medication. This may not be an earth-shattering realization, but the point is, why start someone on medication if they can get through their troubles without it, particularly when one considers the very serious effects that medications can have.

Case Example

An interesting situation concerning medication occurred at Burch House when we admitted a man who had been placed into a Veterans Affairs hospital after having had several psychotic episodes. While in the hospital, he was heavily medicated, and doctors told him he would have to take the medications for the rest of his life. This man had been a marine in Vietnam, and his psychosis appeared to be a posttraumatic reaction. When he first came to Burch House, he rapidly withdrew from the medication he had been taking for 5 months. He could do this because his doctor had allowed him to be responsible for his own medication.

His withdrawal progressed well, without any symptoms occurring for 6 months. After that, he flew into a wild psychosis in which he became a soldier protecting Burch House from the enemy. He would crawl on his belly in and around the house and stay up all night on constant guard against intruders. He was a strong man and sometimes liked to control the people and situations around him forcefully. Although he would occasionally squeeze an arm or pull somebody with him to the next room or onto the couch, he never hurt anyone. At Burch House, things continued around him as normally as possible under the circumstances.

One evening, after 5 days and sleepless nights, this man asked a staff member to give him one of his haloperidol pills so that he could sleep. After a long restful night, he woke up without psychosis. I have been in touch with this man regularly since he left Burch House 6 years ago, and he has never had another breakdown and has never been on medication since that one pill over 6 years ago.

This point of view about medication use presupposes that an emotional breakdown or upheaval is a process that has a beginning and an end. It also presupposes that, through crisis intervention and/or family or couples therapy, a major illness can be circumvented. It assumes that mental illness is socially determined rather than biologically caused. I am not blaming the parents, teachers, or society. I know how difficult it can be to raise children, particularly when the children are difficult themselves. I know how difficult life can be—to earn a living and to survive. I know that just trying to get through life often involves pain and suffering that may seem unbearable, not to mention the anger, greed, and unfairness of life. I am not interested in blaming anyone; I am only interested in solutions that do not harm anyone in the process. Sometimes medications and treatment do a lot of harm and little good. Those are the situations I would like to see avoided. The real point here has very little to do with the "cause" or "treatment" of emotional distress per se, but rather with the options that exist for people in distress or crisis, regardless of how serious—options that are not the mainstream medical approach to treatment or philosophy.

Admission Criteria

When Burch House opened, we were willing to accept virtually anybody, and, in fact, we did. We admitted alcoholic, suicidal, psychotic, anxious, depressed, destructive, manipulative, borderline individuals and almost anyone who was not actively trying to kill themselves or someone else. We sometimes had two or three psychotic people at the same time. This is in a house in which only up to eight patients and four interns live, and people's moods and behaviors bounce from one person to the next like electricity. At times, we had someone at Burch House with multiple diagnoses.

A patient who wants to come to Burch House can simply write or telephone to arrange an interview. Initially, a potential patient visits one afternoon for an hour or two and meets as many members of the community as possible. Generally, we have a group meeting with the prospective patient and then give him or her a tour of the house. After at least a few days have passed, the prospective patient is invited back as our guest for a 3-day visit. During those 3 days, we usually have another group meeting. Hopefully, the nature of Burch House is conveyed and we each get a good sense of one another so we can make a decision with the potential patient. Sometimes our patients come from very far away, and, in those situations, we forego the initial phase of the interview and begin with the 3-day visit. In both instances we require that the prospective patient leave Burch House after the interview for at least a day while we make our part of the decision.

We do not have an ideal patient in mind when we consider someone for Burch House. Our basic consideration is that the individual wants to come and is willing to participate in the activities and care of the household. There is room for all sorts of people at Burch House with different values and ways of doing things. The people of Burch House are generally quite open and accepting of who other people are. We are not homophobic, and we are sensitive to feminist issues and the issues of being a man in our society. We do not believe that we have the answers to life's questions and that there is a right way that one can decide for another. One thing we can do for each other is to help find the possibilities that exist given who we are and who we could possibly be.

Case Example

Very early in our history we took on an 18-year-old woman who the emergency on-call worker of the local mental health clinic brought to us. The on-call worker had given Ms. S. the option of coming to Burch House or going into a hospital. Ms. S. was psychotic, very talkative, and frightened. Her psychosis had the quality of an LSD trip from which she was not coming down. For the most part, except for brief periods of being frightened, she seemed to be having a wonderful time painting the walls of her room, seemingly seeing things and understanding things about her life she had not experienced before. We had to stay with Ms. S. 24 hours a day during her psychosis.

Often, she would want us to keep her in her room while she struggled to get out. These periods of struggle and wrestling always were followed by a period of calm. I believed that symbolically she was struggling to get through or out of being stuck in her psychotic state. If we kept her contained in the room then the struggle was internal, whereas running out of the room would allow her to escape from the internal struggle. Ms. S. cleared from her psychosis in less than 2 weeks.

We realized that her psychosis was triggered by an overdose of amphetamines that she had been using regularly, along with marijuana and alcohol. Ms. S. had had a more serious overdose experience about 2 years earlier, which almost killed her. She had recently abandoned her 10-month-old child because the responsibility was too great, and she was afraid she was too abusive. During her years at Burch House, we found out that she had been the victim of sexual abuse from her father and that she had a very serious addiction to alcohol. It took Ms. S. nearly 4 years of intensive work to feel stable enough to successfully make it in the world. She is currently in a stable marriage, has a young child, and works as a staff member in a group home.

This situation had multiple or complex diagnoses, because of the addiction to alcohol and amphetamines coupled with the psychosis and abusive history. We no longer take on people who are addicted to alcohol or drugs. We learned the hard way how difficult it is to control access to these substances in an open environment like Burch House. Although it is obvious that the addiction is intricately bound to the whole complexity of the problem, it is important to be free of these substances before the emotional work can be done in earnest. I did not always think this way, but after trying many times to work with people as they struggled with or gave in to their addiction, I believe it is a waste of time.

Discussion

I have described only two of the stories about Burch House to illustrate what we are. Regardless of the cases I cited, we have only worked with a small percentage of psychotic individuals. We have been with many people through a variety of crisis situations and struggles through difficult processes. More than 100 patients have come and gone since we started. About 25% have had some type of psychotic episode either at Burch House or before they came there. Many people who came to Burch House had depression and severe anxiety and had been sexually abused early in their lives. It is difficult to say which type of patient is best served by Burch House, but I believe that this type of facility works well for people who have not yet been hospitalized or medicated.

Only about 50% of our patients have ever used medication. In some situations, people could not withdraw from medication at Burch House, after trying repeatedly. Many never even entertained the idea of stopping their medication. It is interesting that anyone who was not on medication did not start taking medication while they were at Burch House.

A small percentage of patients at Burch House were never appropriate for us nor we for them. Although we believe that more than one-half of the patients who have come and gone from Burch House have benefited a great deal, some benefited very little, and a few harbor angry feelings toward us. I imagine that this is experienced in any facility.

Many people believe that someone else is going to heal them or cure them. I do not believe that there are any saviors in the field of psychology, and thinking that there are creates expectations and unrealistic and potentially harmful hierarchies. Therapists, like patients, are ordinary people with their own troubles and relative levels of maturity. I think we must do our best to be present, honest, and responsible—patients as well as therapists.

Cost

Burch House has always prided itself with having probably the lowest fee in the United States for a private psychiatric residential facility. At present our fee is $85 per day, and there are no extra costs except for long-distance phone calls. A lot of small, hidden extras are contained in the fee such as going to the movies, to shows, or to concerts as a group. We are not eligible to receive third-party reimbursement, so patients must pay our fee. Although we have done a lot of charity work, it has been more difficult to raise outside money in recent years, so the fee has become more important.

Philosophy

Burch House is a dwelling, a household, a community of people resting or searching, perhaps at peace or deeply troubled. The beauty of a therapeutic community is that it provides a chance to live one's life in the presence of others who are participants rather than onlookers. Therapy is not something that is done to a patient; it is a dialogue that redefines the negative images we hold on to and that leads to growth, opportunity, and going forward in life. People spend real time with one another and give room for true expression of the heart, the soul, the spirit, and the mind.

Burch House, both as a facility and an idea, is an evolutionary process, which is far from complete. The people of Burch House have been pioneering an approach to practical psychotherapy that is relatively unknown in the United States. There has been very little by way of example to fall back on. In our 14 years we have gained a lot of experience through trial and error. I think our experience has taught a lot more about what not to do than what we should do. The real point is that it provides a choice for people in trouble.

At the start of Burch House I was under the mistaken assumption that we could help people by some way other than being participants in a person's process within a relatively open, honest setting. It has taken a lot of difficult and sometimes painful lessons to realize that one cannot do something to or for another person to make them well, but that people must learn to help themselves. In fact, I believe that supporting the notion that one can "fix" another perpetuates an illusion and fantasy that can lead to trouble.

Those of us who practice in the field of psychotherapy in the United States do so in an atmosphere that holds the practitioner responsible for the actions and manipulations of her or his patient (Schaef 1992). This strips individuals of responsibility for their own actions, and leads to viewing the therapist as someone above human frailty. In addition, our practice is often dictated by an insurance industry whose values and interests are those of businesswomen and men and not those of the practitioners and consumers of the system they represent.

We are all influenced by our own value systems, and it is rare to be able to see these influences at work. Experts in our world are very important, because they can impart a great deal of helpful knowledge. However, care must be taken that decisions are not made for others based on our values in the name of expertise, or an elitist class is created. This is precisely what R. D. Laing (1960, 1967, 1985) was against, and it is the origin of the term *antipsychiatry*. Laing hoped that the practice of true psychiatry did not contain the inherent dangers of a value-laden system that could harm people. I am not talking here about the issue of medication. Laing told me that he had never been opposed to biological psychiatrists, but rather to psychoanalysts who put people in diagnostic categories from a stance of subjective prejudice.

It is difficult for me to write about this work without being concerned about how we treat each other. Distress and serious suffering could happen anywhere, any time, to anyone. The principles of humanity, compassion, morality, and a strong sense of what I would want for myself or my loved ones if we were in trouble, have guided Burch House's development.

The consumers, the practitioners, the third-party payers, and the legislators—all of us—are caught in this same system of expectation, expertise, and quick-fix solutions for problems that need time, space, and open-hearted wisdom. But the good news is that, from the conversations I have been having with colleagues, and new things I am reading, I believe that our profession is beginning to realize this. Changes are being made that may give new direction to the human sciences (McNamee and Gergen 1992; Schaef 1992). The time is right for facilities such as Burch House to start up on their own or in conjunction with existing mental health systems to offer an alternative to current treatment options.

Many fears and superstitions surround mental illness and emotional distress. There are also true stories of terrible things done by emotionally unstable people, and, for this reason, hospitals are necessary. Most people who are lost, suffering, or confused are trying to get home. A homelike environment has a more positive impact on the healing process than being locked in a building away from one's familiar support and surroundings. The therapeutic community provides this environment in a compassionate, simple, and cost-effective manner.

Conclusion

In this chapter I have written about something I love; something that has taught me a great deal and has changed my life. This work has exposed me to much of the pain and joy in life. Being with others struggling to find themselves and their reasons for living has helped me to find my reasons for living life to its fullest, through work, family, home, friends, gardening, and music; wherever the richness of life can be found. It has helped me to realize the importance of getting on with life rather than dwelling on the negative aspects of it. This work cannot be done alone but only by people working together. I encourage others to pursue the therapeutic community as a way to be with people in distress, for it is here that one can find meaning and depth.

References

Barnes M, Berke J: Mary Barnes: Two Accounts of a Journey Through Madness. New York, Harcourt Brace Jovanovich, 1972

Cooper R: Thresholds Between Philosophy and Psychoanalysis: Papers From the Philadelphia Association. New York, Columbia University Press, 1989

Laing RD: The Divided Self. New York, Pantheon, 1960

Laing RD: The Politics of Experience. New York, Pantheon, 1967

Laing RD: Wisdom, Madness and Folly: The Making of a Psychiatrist. London, Macmillan, 1985

McNamee S, Gergen K (eds): Therapy as Social Construction. London, Sage, 1992

Mosher LR, Menn A: Community residential treatment for schizophrenia: two-year follow-up data. Hosp Community Psychiatry 24:391–395, 1978

Schaef AW: Beyond Therapy, Beyond Science: A New Model for Healing the Whole Person. San Francisco, CA, Harper, 1992

The Windhorse Program for Recovery

Editor's Note

FACULTY AND GRADUATES OF THE EAST-WEST PSYCHOLOGY PROGRAM of the Naropa Institute, a Buddhist college in Boulder, Colorado, developed the treatment approach outlined in this chapter. The Windhorse program is about as noninstitutional as the treatment of acute psychosis can be. The disturbed person lives in his or her own home and is helped by a team of people who join the patient in various daily activities. Some may be live-in housemates, and others may join the patient to play basketball or chess, to go for hikes, or to talk about politics or spiritual issues. Throughout, there is an underlying sense of the benefit of human contact, the value in "being with" the patient rather than "doing things to" him or her, and an emphasis on patience and empathy. As in several of the programs in this section of the book, an attempt is made to keep the use of antipsychotic medication to a minimum, with hope that the healing nature of the environment will change the course of the patient's illness.

Chapter 10

The Windhorse Program for Recovery

Jeffrey M. Fortuna, M.A.

*T*he Windhorse program for recovery provides individually designed and comprehensive treatment for psychologically disturbed people in home environments. This innovative program was described by its founder, Edward M. Podvoll, M.D., in *The Seduction of Madness* (1990). This book presents a whole-person view of psychosis and recovery that is illuminated by first-hand reports and the author's clinical experience. Dr. Podvoll described the methods of compassionate care, which involve a team of skilled therapists working closely with a disturbed person in his or her own home. The network of these individual treatment households, together with the households of the staff members, have formed an extended therapeutic community. This community was initially established in Boulder, Colorado, in 1981 and has expanded to Halifax, Nova Scotia, Canada, in 1989 and to Northampton, Massachusetts, in 1992, where I am the director of Windhorse Associates, Inc.

Principles of Theory and Method

The following are the four essential principles at Windhorse:

1. *Psychosis is a major disruption in the balance of the body-mind-environment system* that dislocates the person from the functional reference points of ordinary life. An effective treatment program must work with all of the imbalances in the biological, psychological, social, and spiritual dimensions of the whole person.
2. *Significant recovery is a real possibility* for anyone with psychosis. The person's intrinsic intelligence continually interrupts any psychotic turbulence with momentary experiences of insight and

171

freshness that bring him or her into more direct contact with his or her body and surroundings. The experience is a coming to one's senses, as if awakening from a dream. Such fragile moments are "islands of clarity" that must be recognized and protected as the seeds of recovery.

3. *Recovery can occur naturally when catalyzed by authentic therapeutic friendships* in a homelike setting. Grouping severely disturbed people together in one place of treatment may risk the health of patients and staff. An ill person is likely to become healthier when in the company of other healthy people in a sane environment.

4. *A Windhorse treatment team attends to the recovery of the patient* and is also committed to the well-being of each team member, the patient's family, and the entire therapeutic community. The traditional meaning of a healing community resides in this wide-ranging intention.

These principles, when contemplated and experienced in clinical practice, can arouse the cheerfulness and resourcefulness required to properly attend to someone on the arduous journey of recovery. This attitude is an antidote to the potential exhaustion of one's compassion and resources and is embodied in the name we chose for our service and community:

> Windhorse refers to a mythic horse, famous throughout central Asia, who rides in the sky and is the symbol of man's energy and discipline to uplift himself. Windhorse is literally an energy in the body and mind, which can be aroused in the service of healing an illness or overcoming depression. (Podvoll 1990, p. 24)

These principles translate into a comprehensive method of care that is simple and effective and that has withstood the test of time.

The method of care used in the Windhorse program is home-based team treatment. The pattern and cost of clinical teams vary on a continuum of intensity, depending on what is needed and the available financial resources. Three primary components comprise an intensive team (a partial team is less elaborate):

1. *Therapeutic household*—with live-in housemate(s); a home setting that is established as the locus of treatment for each patient

2. *Basic attendance*—a specialized form of therapeutic relationship that is provided by a team leader and several team therapists
3. *Intensive psychotherapy*—provided by a principal therapist in individual therapy sessions

To supplement the skills of the core team, adjunctive services may be useful. A psychiatrist most often joins each team to monitor medications or to provide psychotherapy. These components will be clarified in the clinical examples to follow.

A pattern of meetings, facilitated by the team leader and principal therapist, integrates the team's activities. These meetings include the weekly team meeting of team members and the patient, which is of central importance; the household meeting in the home with the patient and his or her roommate(s); the team leader's meeting with the principal therapist; the supervision meeting with team therapists; and family meetings with the patient and his or her family members. If several therapeutic homes are in operation, then additional meetings include a community meeting of all therapists and patients; an all-staff meeting; and housemate meetings of past and present roommates. These larger meetings are often held in team members' homes and provide opportunities to socialize. This meeting pattern gives structural coherence to the treatment situation and avoids the fragmentation in care and impersonal relations often found in situations with multiple care providers. These meetings form a matrix of social containment that is essential because no fixed facility provides a physical boundary to the therapeutic environment.

The core clinical group organizes the household and the team. They assess the patient's needs, capacities, and available financial resources, in consultation with the patient and his or her family. An affordable treatment prescription is then tailored to the patient's situation by combining more or less of each of the primary and adjunctive components and the types of meetings. This design adapts to the uniquely evolving situation of the patient, and future adjustments are made in collaboration with the patient and family. Each team is intended to decrease in size and cost over time, although the patient's social involvement with the Windhorse therapeutic community is encouraged after formal treatment has ended. We openly acknowledge the possibility of significant recovery, but do not predict the degree or direction the recovery may take. In practice, we commit ourselves to be in empathic contact with the patient's present condition and life situation.

The forms of a Windhorse team are as varied as the range of patients' unique life situations. Our experience has shown that the most stable recovery from psychotic imbalance occurs in the familiar surroundings of one's home attended by gentle companions.

Case Examples

Below I describe one intensive team and two partial teams to illustrate the principles of the Windhorse theory and method. Consideration has been given to confidentiality.

Case 1

I was referred by a colleague to the director of the rural treatment center in Europe where Jonah had been a resident for 3 years. Jonah had made progress recovering from disabling chronic schizophrenia and was now able to minimally perform tasks of daily living and to communicate with others. The director and Jonah's family believed that a highly structured therapeutic environment in an urban setting would foster his maturity. Jonah wanted relief from a relentlessly tormenting "voice" that for 5 years had caused "heavy feelings" in his "soul." He also wanted to live independently and to someday visit India.

I contracted with a team leader, and we negotiated program cost and design with Jonah's parents and the referring director. We invited Jonah to visit us for a week in Nova Scotia for a "mutual interview" (Fortuna 1987). Before the visit, a psychiatrist, three team therapists, and a potential housemate joined us to form the initial team. When I hire a team member, I ask myself, "Would I want to be with this person if I were ill and unable to care for myself?" We had several meetings to prepare ourselves for the visit and to design a schedule of clinical and social events that would give Jonah sample experiences of the program. During the visit, Jonah expressed, despite his withdrawal and the language barrier, his desire to be free of the "voice" and to be more independent. Jonah was appropriate for our program because he was nonviolent, could safely spend time alone and relate to a schedule, was personally motivated to come, and had cognitive ability and talents.

Jonah presents himself as a 30-year-old self-absorbed man. His current therapist informed us that Jonah often inspires other people to feel affection toward him even though he offers so little of himself in return. Jonah's face is obscured by brown, bushy eyebrows, a full beard, and long hair that drapes his cheeks and neck. His skin is pallid and lackluster. His stocky frame of medium height is slouched and rigid with atrophied muscle tone. Jonah tends to neglect personal hygiene, and his dark-colored clothes are unkempt. When left alone he sinks into himself in bed for long periods. He can exhibit a surprising precision in the way he handles an object or shakes someone's hand. He mutters semiaudibly to himself in a snarling, exasperated tone, in his mother tongue, "Let me alone! Go away! It's all bullshit!," although he explains that this is the "voice" speaking through him. He has an addictive preference for caffeine, nicotine, alcohol, or street drugs, which intensify his symptoms. He has been relatively stable for the past 2 years on 4 mg/day of haloperidol (Haldol), although he is unhappy with the drug's side effects. Jonah's eyes are clear gray-blue, and he usually has a fixed, downcast gaze, although he often makes prolonged, startling eye contact. After long moments, he and I would usually smile together, exchange a few words, and look away. This contact illuminates Jonah's aura of angry impenetrability and conveys the impression of a person of significant depth of feeling and intelligence who is both drawn to and terrified of human relationships.

The Program

- *Household:* Jonah resided with a male housemate in a rented, modestly furnished 2-bedroom home in a quiet residential neighborhood during his 14 months in Nova Scotia. The housemate and Jonah spent several hours together each day in ordinary domestic living, sharing responsibility for housework and cooking. Weekly household meetings were facilitated by the team leader to review necessary chores, the arrangement of the environment, the household budget, relationships between house members, and plans for hosting guests. Naturally, the dirts of soiled air and floors, of unspoken resentments, and of depression accumulated in the environment. However, we reminded each other of the slogan, "Train in cleaning up after yourself," as a bedrock ecological effort for maintaining a decent household.
- *Basic attendance:* Four team therapists and the team leader individually attended to Jonah during 3-hour shifts in his home and in the field.

Two shifts were scheduled each weekday, and one 6-hour shift was scheduled each weekend day to allow for leisurely excursions into the countryside. On this particular team, the therapists had master's degrees in clinical psychology, with extensive clinical experience. They also trained in a type of mindfulness-awareness meditation that reveals the common tendency to be absorbed in habitual patterns of thinking. This experience allowed the therapists to have deeper empathy with Jonah's entrapment in mental projection. Mindfulness-awareness practice provides the therapists with personal knowledge of how one's body and mind can be joined and synchronized, which is also the intent of basic attendance. The quiet household setting provided opportunities for team members to attend to Jonah by gently encouraging him to refocus his distracted attention on the sensory details of ordinary activities. By practicing these "domestic disciplines" (Fortuna 1987), Jonah strengthened his concentration and knit his mind, body, and environment more closely together. Contemplative practices are relied on by increasing numbers of therapists to coordinate the body and mind as the foundation of personal health and of the healing relationship (see, for example, Kabat-Zinn 1990).

Four adjunctive team members had weekly contact with Jonah: a language tutor, an acupuncture and massage practitioner, a psychiatric nurse, and a psychiatrist who monitored Jonah's medication and general health. Each adjunctive person attends a monthly team meeting.

- *Intensive psychotherapy (IP):*   As the principal therapist, I met with Jonah during four 1-hour sessions per week in the formal setting of an office. IP is a specialized form of basic attendance rooted in the tradition of Edward Podvoll, Harold Searles, Otto Will, Frieda Fromm-Reichmann, and Harry Stack Sullivan. The basic premise of IP is that human intimacy is a significant catalyst for recovery from psychosis. IP aims to cultivate an authentic therapeutic friendship. "Authentic" means to recognize that empathy with the patient's experience happens naturally as the starting point. "Therapeutic" means to search for and give proper voice to the truth available in every interpersonal moment. "Friendship" means that the patient and therapist become trusted companions who encourage each other in a process of mutual learning. In the Windhorse approach, the principal therapist is just one element in an integrated treatment network, rather than the single point of meaningful therapeutic contact.

The root interpersonal discipline of basic attendance can appear deceptively simple in its focus on ordinary daily activities and on simply being with Jonah. It involves many degrees of sophistication to properly attend to the intricate function of synchronizing mind with body and environment without forcing a particular outcome. It is the concerted effort of the group of people who practice basic attendance— with the patient and with each other—that constitutes the work of the healing team. This is not a conventional multidisciplinary group of specialists, such as a psychiatrist, social worker, or nurse, who some- times consult together about their individual work with a patient. Rather, it is a team that is facilitated by on-site leaders, internally accountable, and whose members are openly responsive to each other and to the task. This type of working team can increasingly be found in the most successful business and political organizations worldwide.

The team leader and I co-lead the weekly team meetings and individ- ually supervise team members. I maintained bimonthly telephone contact with Jonah's father, who became a close collaborator in the treatment. I worked with Jonah's team 10 hours per week. The team leader works 15 hours per week supervising the household, especially the housemate, and tracks the details of program budget, schedule, and case management. We are available to the team 24 hours a day by telephone.

Jonah's program cost $300 per day. This provided flexible and comprehensive treatment for Jonah's unique life predicament in his own home, far below the cost of hospital care.

The journey of treatment. The daily schedule provided a pre- dictable structure that safely moved the healing environment forward. The precision of the schedule sharpened Jonah's and the team members' awareness of the boundaries of experience, such as between work and relaxation, or between daydreaming and attending to the situation at hand. To be alone for long periods drifting into the future is unhealthy for any person recovering from psychosis, especially from the negative symptoms of lack of motivation, blunted affect, and social withdrawal. Constant attention to a schedule was the background of our work with Jonah.

The weekday schedule for Jonah was typically as follows:

8 A.M.:   Awakened by housemate or alarm; Jonah tried to dress and to attend to hygiene.

9 A.M. to Noon: Team therapist helped Jonah with dressing and hygiene, if needed, and to tidy the bedroom; prepared breakfast, ate together, and cleaned up; took medication; reviewed daily checklist for morning routine; did preassigned house chores together; remained at home or engaged in an outside activity such as walking, shopping, or going to the library, a cafe, or a class; rode bus alone to IP appointment.

12–12:50 P.M.:   IP session.

1–1:30 P.M.:   Rode bus or walked home alone.

1:30–3:30 P.M.:   Attended language tutorial or session with acupuncture and massage therapist, or rested at home alone.

3:30–6:30 P.M. (less structured than morning shift):   Engaged in an outside activity with team therapist; remained at home and conversed, read, or listened to music; prepared dinner, ate, and cleaned up together, with housemate; took medication.

Evening: Spent time with housemate or alone; went to bed after dinner or stayed up later (regular bedtime encouraged).

The first spring.   The fresh beginning with Jonah's arrival was reflected in the bright skies and flowers of spring. The team attended to the practicalities of establishing the household and to developing rapport with Jonah. We gently urged Jonah to participate despite his well-honed resistance to intrusion by us or the "voice." Each person, with word, touch, or gesture, began to gently call Jonah's attention back from distraction. We observed that Jonah compulsively ate unprepared food, smoked cigarettes, paced, muttered incessantly, and lay prone for long periods drifting in and out of trance, dream, and sleep. Organizing healthier life rhythms was the first priority. An irregularity in Jonah's cardiac pulse was corrected by improving diet, exercise, and rest; by reducing the haloperidol by 50%; and by massage and acupuncture. Jonah alternated between passive compliance and stubborn resistance to these changes in life-style. The team acknowledged the risks of this exercise of therapeutic power, for example, in possibly reinforcing Jonah's sense of persecution. They explained to Jonah the practical necessity of such protective boundaries and that our primary intention was to encourage his personal motivation and independence. Jonah's English was barely adequate, which further strained interpersonal contact and increased his sense of alienation. The concerted efforts of Jonah and the team to learn each other's languages became the tangible model for communicating through his isolation.

The task for the IP sessions was for Jonah and me to learn to meaningfully communicate. We settled down in long silences and often shared a cup of tea. I had to abandon strategies to change or rescue Jonah to truly listen to him. Frieda Fromm-Reichmann (1959) taught that the one prerequisite for all intensive psychotherapy is: "The therapist must be able to listen . . . in this other person's own right" (p. 65). IP is a controversial aspect of the Windhorse approach. Most psychiatrists with whom I have spoken have assured me that such intensive therapy is too stimulating for the fragilely defended ego, is an anachronism now that we have biomedical science and neuroleptics, has not been shown by research to be of benefit, is not cost-effective, and has only been useful in elucidating psychotic phenomenology. Critics often fail to appreciate that IP acquires unique value when practiced within an integrated therapeutic team. I am also faced with personal doubts that nothing is really happening, that I am not trained enough to deal with transference issues, or that too much time and money is being spent on just sitting together. During a session, Jonah, with a word or glance, drew me out of these moments of doubt back to our relational space. Jonah was always on time for our sessions, and we both valued our time together.

I introduced an exercise to help Jonah control his involuntary muttering and snarling that was distracting us. Sitting side by side, we focused our attentions on a clock for 2-minute intervals and held our mouths closed, breathing normally. During the exercise, Jonah's mouth did not move, and, to his surprise, he reported that he did not hear the "voice." Later, the practice was transferred to the shifts, and the interval was extended to 5 minutes. Eventually, Jonah learned to hold his mouth still and to stop the "voice" for several minutes at will, enabling him to stabilize and extend these islands of clarity.

In the second month, we celebrated Jonah's birthday, the team leader's new pregnancy, and a housewarming at the household with the team members' families. Jonah's anxiety and repressed anger were more apparent, and we had a healthy respect for how he might eventually express his emotions.

The summer. This is the season of growth and activity. Jonah became more alive to the world around him, evidenced by a flushed complexion, robust movements, and clearer eyes. He briefly attended pottery lessons, where he angrily pounded clay and smashed discarded pots. Often he was in a rage with agitated, restless movements and occasionally experienced sleepless nights. Team members experienced sharper alternations in being in and out of contact with Jonah. The structure in the household was increased (e.g., Jonah had to be fully clothed at home and could not smoke in his bedroom), which further irritated him. The housemate became uneasy, and he and the team leader were in conflict. The housemate gave notice that he would resign in the fall, and we began to doubt our decision to staff the household with only one roommate. The situation seemed directionless and potentially unsafe, and this seemed to mirror Jonah's experience. The team banded more tightly together by emphasizing precision of schedule and communication.

The tension increased prior to Jonah's parents' week-long visit to Nova Scotia in the fifth month. During a team meeting with Jonah and his parents, we agreed that Jonah was waking up in the middle of his nightmare with no apparent means of escape, while experiencing his pain more clearly. Jonah's mother explained that he had been at this point on three past occasions, "but he always ran away before and now he cannot run away." They could not agree to his request to live with them, and Jonah became increasingly agitated. We discussed with Jonah what he needed in his life. We agreed to allow him to smoke in his room if he used an air purifier and smoke alarms, to have freer use of pocket money, and to begin to plan a vacation for him and a team member. Jonah's mother stated that "a person must have a vision," and if Jonah's was to visit India, then we could build on that interest in every imaginable way. Later, we gently encouraged his parents to abandon feelings of guilt of having failed as parents. We emphasized that their present mental health had a positive impact on Jonah and the team. The morning of their departure, Jonah was very sad and despondent; his eyes welled with tears. Long gazes between Jonah and team members seemed laden with loneliness.

The autumn. The pace of summer slowed to the cool season of harvest. Jonah became more withdrawn and depressed, and he began to ignore the schedule. This regression coincided with his parents' departure, the roommate's termination, a change in language tutors, and the team leader's increasing introversion with her pregnancy. Jonah's haloperidol was increased, and diazepam (Valium) was prescribed. (Note: over 14 months of treatment, haloperidol was adjusted across a range of 1–5 mg/day, and diazepam was adjusted across a range of 5–20 mg/day.) This had a positive effect, which was reinforced when we hired a roommate who was the same age as Jonah. He had a natural affinity for being with eccentric people and was a student of the healing arts. Soon after moving in, the roommate revealed, to our surprise, that he was 4 months into his recovery from severe drug use. The team became trusted elders to him, and he grew significantly over the next year. Jonah's and the roommate's parallel journeys of recovery served to strengthen their camaraderie.

Jonah became curious about the smallest details of things, whether the name and origin of a particular tea or the place where a team member grew up. He began using a fragrant cologne and enjoying luxurious bubble baths. He attended the cinema with steady attention and resumed weekly swimming lessons that he had begun the previous summer. He began to report that the "voice" could now "taste what I taste, hear what I hear, feel what I feel." This may have been the beginning reintegration of Jonah and the projected "other." We began to remind Jonah of decent manners, such as in addressing other people or in eating a meal. Behaving with respect toward one's environment uplifts a person from the obliviousness that degrades body and mind.

By December's end, Jonah's psychotic agitation and withdrawal increased, because he felt the emptiness of being away from home for the holidays. He spent Christmas day at my home with family and friends, remaining anxiously withdrawn on the periphery.

The winter. The sun was at its lowest point, and Jonah longed for a warmer, brighter climate. His frustration and loneliness mounted to an acute psychotic episode. One morning he had a barber cut his beard and hair short, and his muttering and movements became pressured in an explosive buildup. In our IP session I was shocked to see his face so exposed as if he had suddenly emerged from hiding. He insisted that his loneliness was intolerable and that he must return to his native country. I was unable to slow the escalation. Later in the day, he vigorously punched the air around him, loudly played rock music, and made unintelligible sounds that frightened his roommate. On an accompanied walk, he pushed a female pedestrian against a parked car, because "she was Canadian," he later reported. She was stunned but unharmed. I met Jonah at the household; he was in bed fully clothed and shaking. I offered him enough medication to reestablish contact. He reiterated his desire to return home, and I agreed to consider this immediately. We remained quietly together into the evening.

The crisis subsided overnight. When Jonah roused from a long, deep sleep, his cognition was stable, his interpersonal contact was excellent, and his motivation to continue with the program was un-ambivalent. The crisis appeared to be an intensification of a charged personal drama to a breaking point, followed by a prolonged island of clarity. The team regards this as a healing crisis. The meaning of the event includes not only Jonah's manifest experience of missing his native language, land, and family, but also his coming into direct contact with his profound loneliness accumulated over years of social withdrawal.

Regarding a psychotic crisis as potentially healing is a mark of an alternative to conventional medical model treatment. The crisis may not be the symptomatic recurrence of a disease once held in remission, requiring suppressive measures for a person to recompensate back to a previous level of functioning. Rather, this may be a crisis of organismic growth initiated by chaotic disintegration of a previously stable state. The crisis is healing if the person reintegrates to a more evolved level of meaning and function; it is destructive if the psychotic disturbance intensifies toward further chaos, injury, or death. The outcome is significantly affected by how one is treated by others and how the person relates to the spontaneously occurring islands of clarity experienced as gaps of doubt and wakefulness in the pressure of the crisis. Gregory Bateson (1961) proposed the notion of a "curative nightmare": "that the body or mind contains, in some form, such wisdom that it can create that *attack* upon itself that will lead to a later resolution of the pathology" (p. xii). Persons in the consumer/survivor movement insist that mental health professionals should consider that a psychotic crisis may have growth potential before altering its vulnerable transitional states with involuntary treatments.

Jonah began to openly describe his depression as "heavy, dark feelings in the soul" that alternated with bright moments of sunlight or the companionship of women. He vacationed in Mexico with his room-mate, curbed his overeating, and reduced his cigarette smoking, all of which made him "feel better and made the 'voice' less difficult." Medications were again reduced. Jonah entered a work-oriented day program for disturbed persons and showed surprising skill in long-neglected hobbies of chess and backgammon. He showed more concern for the team members, frequently offering tea on shifts. A major focus for the remaining months became learning conversation skills. We began planning for Jonah's departure, although it had been decided, with his input, that he would stay for an additional 2 months.

The second spring. The cycle of the seasons has been completed. The team relaxed the program structure and gave Jonah more responsibility (e.g., having unsupervised pocket money), which communicated that he could care for himself. Increasingly, he was attentive to his surroundings and made poignant attempts at conversation. He was "coming out" with the tentative awkwardness of one emerging from a harrowing inner ordeal. The team members expressed sadness as our team community prepared to disband. Jonah would join a partial Windhorse-style team in a familiar European town, accompanied by his current roommate who would continue to live with him.

We had a weekly team meeting the day before the second birthday celebration for Jonah, 2 weeks before he was to leave Nova Scotia. His psychotic turmoil had intensified over the past 48 hours. Amidst forceful vocalizations and facial contortions, he complained of the relentless torture of the "voice," of his inability to do anything for himself, and of his wish to die. The team offered him empathic reassurances and the obvious termination-anxiety interpretation to no avail. He insisted that we did not understand him, nor he us, and that there was no hope for him. With no way to bridge the abyss with Jonah, the team doubted its work of the past year. I remembered, with some comfort, that at the end of anyone's treatment, the entire original problem often recycles as if nothing useful had happened. I decided to delay sharing this conceptual interpretation, as I believed to do so would drain the life out of this poignant group experience. The meeting ended with no resolution.

The following morning Jonah was pleased to awaken to birthday phone calls from both parents. The birthday celebration was a communal island of clarity, alive with music, children's voices, and good cheer that eased our previous day's struggle with isolation. Jonah responded with smiles to the thoughtful gifts and affectionate farewells that he received.

After 14 months together, the team met at the household. A photo album of Jonah and the team was presented to Jonah. Final good-byes and well-wishes were exchanged, and then it was time for Jonah and the roommate to leave. The team stayed for a final cleaning of the house, and then disbanded.

I have remained in contact with Jonah, his parents, and his roommate in Europe. Jonah has continued his slow, steady recovery in the context of a small therapeutic team and household. He and his roommate have plans for the long-sought visit to India. Jonah's parents and others who knew him before the Windhorse experience acknowledge his improving health.

Case 2

Rich's parents were referred to our service by the staff of a psychiatric hospital where Rich, age 30, had been a patient for 2 months and was soon to be discharged. The authorities had removed him from his parents' home and had taken him to the hospital during an acute episode of a disorder previously diagnosed as "schizoaffective." After meeting with the hospital staff, the family, and Rich, I agreed that Rich would live alone in an apartment supported by social assistance and continue under the care of his psychiatrist of 7 years, to be paid by medical insurance. A team leader, myself as the principal therapist, and three team therapists would compose the therapeutic team. Rich would learn to live independently by developing his interests, a career, and a social life outside of the family circle.

Each team therapist and the team leader met with Rich twice per week for 3-hour shifts of basic attendance, totaling eight shifts per week. I met with Rich for two weekly IP sessions and joined Rich and his psychiatrist monthly to discuss medications. Rich spent Sundays at his parents' home. The psychiatrist, cognizant of the danger of tardive dyskinesia, was currently eliminating Rich's haloperidol and phasing in buspirone (BuSpar), an antianxiety agent. I met weekly with the team leader for planning and supervision, and we met monthly with Rich's parents, most often including Rich. Supervision of the team members occurred in team meetings and by telephone. The cost of the service to the family began at $130 per day, decreasing to $30 per day currently as Rich's capabilities have strengthened. These figures do not reflect housing and psychiatrist costs. My leaving and that of another team member reduced the team's size and cost and transferred more responsibility to Rich. Rich continues to attend the weekly 1-hour team meetings, now more central to the integration of the smaller team.

A key clinical issue had been Rich's proper emancipation from home. During a recent "paranoid episode," Rich reported that he actually was barricaded in his bedroom to give him the privacy to plan how to move out, while his parents were privately discussing the same matter. There has been no overt sign of psychotic disturbance since Rich began with the team. A year later, Rich has become a trusted elder in the family matrix, modeling the process of leaving home for the younger siblings. The family has matured, and Rich has discovered the necessary courage to relate more truthfully with himself and others. Despite his shyness, Rich has become an active participant in the Windhorse community meetings. Rich was not as disturbed as Jonah and thus did not require that degree of care and expense. The journey of the team with Rich was as personally engaging, although not as dramatic, as the experience with Jonah. The current plan is to formally end treatment at the end of the second year, although informal relations between Rich and the Windhorse community will continue.

Case 3

After a lecture I gave on the Windhorse program, an elderly woman approached me and described the condition of her daughter, Kathy. Kathy, now in her 40s, had been suffering since age 18 with a disturbance diagnosed as "chronic paranoid schizophrenia" that had required extensive inpatient care and multiple medications. She had not been able to settle in supervised residential settings and was living with her parents again. Life in the household had deteriorated into intolerable conflict, and her father's heart condition was worsening with the stress. Her parents felt that, unless she had a support network by the time they died, Kathy would succeed with the final in a series of suicide attempts.

A team leader and I met weekly with the family members in their home to mediate conflicts and to establish productive living patterns. The team leader provided case management and one 3-hour shift of basic attendance weekly. She was in almost daily telephone contact with Kathy and her parents as a result of frequent crises. We soon moved to my office for weekly team meetings, with Kathy attending on alternate weeks. The team leader continued with the house meetings.

I met weekly with the team leader for planning and supervision. Kathy's psychiatrist of 20 years, paid by medical insurance, agreed to our involvement if we did "not provide psychotherapy or meddle with the medications." Kathy also used these medicines in attempts to overdose. We agreed, and the psychiatrist has since rescinded both constrictions. The cost for the team was a reduced fee of $13 per day to her parents, because they were living on a small retirement pension.

After 8 months, Kathy moved to an apartment supported by a social service agency with whom the team formed a collaborative relationship. The team expanded to include a student and the director of Kathy's housing agency, who were working as volunteer team therapists with Kathy for their own professional development. Kathy grew into a capable householder and continued to slowly untangle delusions from accurate perceptions with her increasingly stable attention and discriminating doubts. On my leaving Nova Scotia, the team leader became the principal therapist, and a new person assumed her role.

The team is established as a viable learning environment for each member. The work with Kathy continues to be rugged and understaffed as a result of insufficient funds. Recently, her allegiance to health had a setback with a near-lethal overdose attempt. The team remained close to Kathy and her parents during her awakening from a comatose state. Kathy continues to inspire her team with delightful eccentricity, humor, and sincerity. She may remain with some form of the team for the rest of her life. Her parents regard the Windhorse team as "a breath of fresh air" and are now enjoying their "golden years" together. I remain in contact with them and the team by telephone and letters.

Distinctive Features and Implications

The Windhorse program for recovery is a viable alternative to contemporary care offered in long-term inpatient and residential settings. Each treatment team provides compassionate in-home care for a person enduring psychosis or its aftereffects, to facilitate his or her recovery of a dignified and meaningful life. In practice, the Windhorse program works with the imbalances in the biological, psychological, social, and spiritual dimensions of the whole person, as illustrated in the three clinical vignettes.

Biological Dimension

The team utilizes a range of physical treatments in addition to psychiatric medications. Medications are used sparingly, intermittently, and for as long as is necessary without committing to long-term maintenance regimens. Care is taken not to cloud the patient's awareness or to excessively blunt the level of arousal in order to maintain optimal learning ability. This orientation is a source of dialogue with each team's attending psychiatrist. Proper diet and behavior are emphasized, and appropriate physical therapies are considered, such as acupuncture, massage, or movement therapy. A schedule patterns healthy rhythms of daily living. Maintaining a clean and uplifted household is essential. Care of the body and the environment, which promotes wellness, is the basis for recovery and the context for the proper use of medication.

Psychological Dimension

Basic attendance fosters the synchronization of the patient's body, mind, and environment, unhinged by mental illness. The forms of basic attendance are individual psychotherapy, practical or ordinary therapy, specialized group meetings, and family work, which are all integrated into a single team for each patient. Gentle and disciplined friendships between staff and patient gradually develop, which bridge the alienation that usually results from the psychotic disturbance, cultural stigma, and rigid professional distance. The patient is able to recover hidden psychological resources of intelligence and courage within himself or herself that are essential in overcoming the fears and self-aggression that shadow any psychotic episode.

Social Dimension

Treatment and recovery are carried out under ordinary life conditions in individual households in the community. Grouping people with psychosis together in one place may risk everyone's health and reinforces stigma. The team attends to the boundary between the patient and the practical tasks of living and working in the larger social world. The same therapists accompany the patient through all stages of recovery, eliminating the stressful transitions patients experience when they are abruptly admitted to and discharged from discrete programs in sequential levels of care. The "revolving door" problem, such as going in and out of the hospital, is lessened because the intensity and cost of the team adapt to the patient's changing condition. The patient and his or her family become active collaborators in the team as a microhealing community, and the benefits of involvement are shared among everyone. This intimacy of mutual caring fosters bonds of human kinship similar to an extended family or clan.

Spiritual Dimension

The Windhorse community does not promote any particular religious doctrine. It does cultivate a field of dialogue in which the broad range of staff and patient experiences can be safely expressed and responded to. Patients repeatedly ask their caregivers to listen, without judgment or denigration, to their cherished spiritual concerns, such as their relationship to good and evil or to the "divine." Compelling glimpses of ultimate meaning always occur in some stage of psychotic disturbance. Similarly, staff may ask to explore the meaning of true compassion or the relationship of their personal spiritual practice to clinical work. Many Windhorse staff and patients have found contemplative disciplines to enhance self-knowing and to widen awareness beyond private concerns. Members of the Windhorse community are attempting to live productively and creatively together, enlivened by a spirit of learning. To engage in healing is traditionally a sacred art that simultaneously attends to the ill person and other community members and reharmonizes the community with the surrounding environment. This perspective joins social ecology and spirituality together in a time-honored way (Knudtson and Suzuki 1992).

Conclusion

The future of mental health care is increasingly driven by the consumers and survivors of conventional treatments that are influenced by the medical model of psychosis as a brain disease best treated with brain medicine. Consumers insist on being offered humane, whole-person treatment alternatives. The medical model was once the promising alternative to outdated treatments, and it is reasonable to assume, since all models have historically proved to be provisional, that future paradigm shifts are inevitable. There are already signs of a transformation of Western medicine "from a narrow biomedical model to a biopsychosocial one" (Barasch 1992, p. 36). American mental health care is now in a crisis of rising costs, inaccessibility to shrinking community services, and increasing reliance on brief crisis hospitalizations and psychiatric medications (Dumont 1992). In addition, the political and economic alliances between the psychopharmaceutical industry and psychiatry are an increasing source of embarrassment to the profession, and the obvious conflicts of interest left unresolved will intensify the crisis. One can certainly rely on the alternatives to any established system in a crisis of transition. However, as with psychosis, whether such outcomes are healing or destructive significantly depends on our actions now.

References

Barasch D: The mainstreaming of alternative medicine. The New York Times Magazine, October 4, 1992, Part 2

Bateson G: Introduction, in Perceval's Narrative: A Patient's Account of His Psychosis, 1830-1832. Edited by Bateson G. Palo Alto, CA, Stanford University Press, 1961, pp i–xxii

Dumont M: Treating the Poor: A Personal Sojourn Through the Rise and Fall of Community Mental Health. Belmont, MA, Dymphna Press, 1992

Fortuna J: Therapeutic households. Journal of Contemplative Psychotherapy 4:49–76, 1987

Fromm-Reichmann F: Psychoanalysis and Psychotherapy. Chicago, IL, University of Chicago Press, 1959

Kabat-Zinn J: Full Catastrophe Living. New York, Delta Publishing, 1990

Knudtson P, Suzuki D: Wisdom of the Elders. Toronto, Canada, Stoddart Publishing, 1992

Podvoll E: The Seduction of Madness. New York, HarperCollins, 1990

Can Interdependent Mutual Support Function as an Alternative to Hospitalization? The Santa Clara County Clustered Apartment Project

Editor's Note

THE AUTHOR OF THIS CHAPTER CONCEIVED AND HELPED TO ESTABLISH
an innovative series of programs at a large mental health
center in California—living communities of people with mental illness, based on mutual support and interdependence.
These communities of clustered apartments were to be assertively nonclinical in style: staff were encouraged to abandon
traditional roles and to become, instead, community organizers. Would these strengthened communities develop ways to
support their members so that hospital admission for patients
with acute psychiatric distress became less necessary? This
was a question that the project organizers were keen to see
answered. As the project took shape, each of the communities
developed in different ways; some were more successful than
others in functioning as an alternative to the hospital. In one
program, community members provided respite care in a crisis
apartment to members who were acutely disturbed. Other
programs were less able to meet the needs of new or established members. The author explores the reasons for this
variation.

Chapter 11

Can Interdependent Mutual Support Function as an Alternative to Hospitalization? The Santa Clara County Clustered Apartment Project

James Mandiberg, L.C.S.W.

*I*n 1987, The Santa Clara County Mental Health Bureau received funding from the Robert Wood Johnson Foundation to convert three staff-centered residential treatment model programs, whose goal was patient independence, to three nonclinical-nonrehabilitation model patient communities based on mutual support and interdependence among patients. Although these communities were not established to act as alternatives to hospitalization, each attempted to do so. In this chapter, I explore why each community made this attempt, how they structured their interventions, how much success they had in serving as an alternative to the hospital, and what their experience might reveal about the ability of mutual support to act as a hospital alternative for people considered to be severely and persistently mentally ill.

Santa Clara County Mental Health System

As a mental health system in the 1980s, Santa Clara County, California, with a population of 1.4 million, had a community support system

I would like to thank Dr. Yvette Sheline and Dr. Lawrence Telles for their review and comments on earlier drafts of this chapter. I would also like to thank the Robert Wood Johnson Foundation, Dr. Leonard Stein, and Dr. Kenneth Meinhardt for their support and encouragement of the CAP projects.

comparable to the rest of the United States. This system included a county acting as a central mental health authority; a continuum of residential treatment, crisis, respite, and subacute programs; a case management system; several assertive community treatment (ACT) model teams; Fountain House model programs; vocational programs based on supported employment concepts; and a range of specialized services for homeless and ethnic populations. In addition, it had a hospital (where patients had an average length of stay of 7 to 10 days) that pursued an aggressive nonhospitalization policy and a number of traditional model community mental health centers (CMHCs).

The county also benefited from a board of supervisors who were sophisticated about and supportive of mental health services, many board-and-care homes, an innovative and assertive family advocacy and support group, and a history of non-county-funded experimental programs, including Soteria House (Mosher and Menn 1979), the original Fairweather project (Fairweather et al. 1969), and the research of Freddolino and colleagues (1989). Despite the extensive range and high quality of the mental health services for the severely mentally ill patients in the county, we continued to experience many of the same problems, including a high level of recidivism, that other areas less rich in mental health resources experienced. This led to a reanalysis of the organization of our services, the organizational features that might be contributing to these problems, and the organizational or program-level response that might be available to mitigate these problems.

The Need for Support Systems

One response to these problems was to reexamine the support system of patients considered to be severely mentally ill. This revealed that the concept of "support system" combined two very distinct types of support: treatment supports and social supports. We found that many treatment and rehabilitation programs functionally served as both treatment programs and social support networks. Even progressive system models like the National Institute of Mental Health's Community Support Program refers to both treatment and social support programs as community supports (Parrish 1989; Stroul 1988; Turner and Shifren 1979; Turner and TenHoor 1978).

Clinical experience and an increasing body of research seem to indicate that all of us, including those patients considered to be severely mentally ill, require permanent and consistent social support networks to maintain satisfying and healthy community lives (Berkman and Syme 1979; Cohen and Syme 1985; Mitchell and Trickett 1980; Pilisuk and Minkler 1980; Sarason et al. 1990). Yet, it is clear that mental health system patients frequently do not have adequate support networks (Cohen and Sokolovsky 1978; Hammer et al. 1978; Morrison and Bellack 1987). In this situation, patients use any support networks that are available, or they use other systems as if they were social support networks.

In the resulting confusion for patients, the positive potential of social supports is subverted, and dependence on professionally provided treatment as a social support is reinforced. Patients begin to rely on treatment services as if they were social supports. Therefore, there was little mystery to patients' recurrent use of the hospital and other professionally provided means of support (Dincin and Witheridge 1982; Harris and Bergman 1988; Moran et al. 1984). Thus, the required model would clearly separate the concept of treatment and rehabilitation services from that of social supports. Social supports would be designed as permanent, with treatment and rehabilitation services available only as needed.

In our review of the mental health system we also found that the organization of the treatment-rehabilitation system helped to destabilize patients. It is well known that patients with symptoms diagnosed as schizophrenia have problems forming and maintaining relationships with people and places. Yet, most mental health systems require patients to frequently change both the people they relate to and the places where they have become comfortable and secure. This is done, for example, by requiring patients in crisis to first move to hospitals, crisis houses, or hospital alternatives and, after some period of time, to move to various residential treatment programs. This moving about may be convenient for the system, but it is not best for the patient. From the patient's perspective, a far better alternative would be to bring different levels of services to the patient, while he or she remains in the same stable and known environment. System reforms like ACT (Jerrell and Teh Wei 1989; Stein and Test 1980, 1985), case management (Anthony et al. 1988; Kanter 1989; Moxley 1989), and supported housing (Hogan and Carling 1992; Randolf et al. 1987; Ridgeway and Zipple 1990) can all be seen as attempts to address the instability of patients resulting from system-induced changes in relationships and places.

Clustered Apartment Model

Although some have explored patient subculture as a neutral phenomenon (Estroff 1981), most mental health programs now regard the patient subculture as negative. Mental health programs and staff discourage patients from socializing, living together, and ultimately working together. It is considered permissible during treatment or rehabilitation, but not as a permanent arrangement. The usually stated goal of "independence" reinforces this. Thus, even proponents of program models whose success is firmly rooted in the interdependent subculture of patients (e.g., the Fountain House model) ultimately posit independence as the goal (Mastboom 1992; Peterson 1978).

The new model that was developed took a very different approach. This model viewed the client subculture as potentially positive and as a means of providing the permanent social supports that the wider culture and community seemed unwilling or unable to do. Thus, the model was based on the simple concept that if a patient community was given the resources and the assistance to form itself on a positive, mutually supportive basis, it could act as a permanent support system. This had the potential to obviate many of the mental health services that were functioning as de facto social supports under the guise of being treatment. For some patients, this included the hospital.

The model used the clustering of the patients' homes as one vehicle for fostering a community. In the ideal model, a patient could walk to any other patient's house within 5 minutes. Community organizers, rather than clinicians, would assist the clients (or community members) in establishing a mutually supportive and interdependent community. This community was to be available to members as long as they needed or wanted it, without regard to clinical or community status (e.g., hospitalization) (Mandiberg 1987; Mandiberg and Telles 1990; Telles 1992).

This model is different from traditional treatment and rehabilitation programs in the following ways:

- It clearly separates social supports from treatment and rehabilitation services and focuses on the social support needs. It also truly regards the social support needs as more basic and more primary than the treatment needs.
- It views independence as a "false goal," and suggests interdependence and mutual support as a more appropriate goal.

- It views client subculture as being potentially positive. Consequently, rather than seeing the clustering of patients only in its system-created negative form of ghettoization, it looks to the positive potential of client subculture to provide necessary social support.
- It relies on the clients themselves to delineate which treatment and rehabilitation services they believe they need from outside the community and which they believe they can provide within the client community. Thus, the model is consistent with the research of Freddolino and associates (1989); clients can either use the standard mental health system services or alternative intracommunity services.

These considerations led to the development of a nontreatment social support model in 1985, which was approved for 4 years of pilot program funding by the Robert Wood Johnson Foundation Mental Health Services Development Grant in 1987 (Mandiberg 1987). This was combined with existing county funding to three social rehabilitation agencies, which converted residential treatment programs into demonstration projects based on this new model. The Clustered Apartment Project (CAP) was implemented at three different sites: an urban site with a capacity for 68 people, a suburban site with a capacity for 73 people, and a rural site, rapidly becoming a suburban community, with a capacity for 90 people. The latter program was also designed to be a bilingual and bicultural program for Latino patients (Mandiberg and Telles 1990; Telles 1992).

Program Descriptions

Program I

Each program site differed in several ways from the ideal program model. As a physical site, Program I, the urban location, was the closest to the ideal. Duplex apartments in a larger housing development were purchased with federal housing funds through a nonprofit community development agency. One of these apartments—the Center of Attention—was reserved for community members who were experiencing crises. A nearby building was rented as a community center and project office. All of the community members lived within several minutes' walk of each other and the community center. Staff were mostly retrained paraprofessionals from the agency's former residential treatment program. As these staff members left, they were replaced by people who did not have clinical experience, including consumers.

New community members were accepted into the community through a two-step community process. First, new members were interviewed by community members. Once a person was accepted as a member of the community, the next step was to find an apartment to move into. Because the living situations were viewed as permanent, existing roommates had the option to accept or reject a new community member as a roommate. This created a potentially awkward situation of being accepted into the community, but not having a place to live. Consequently, this tended to screen out from community membership people who were seen as potentially having trouble finding roommates; more symptomatic patients were excluded in favor of those seen as less disturbing to the status quo. Thus, the community comprised people considered to have severe and persistent mental illnesses, including a history of high use of intensive mental health services. However, at entry to the program, they tended to be the more clinically stable applicants.

Program II

Program II, the rural/new suburban site, varied from the ideal model in two ways. First, this community's apartments were divided between two small cities about 10 miles apart. However, in each city, the apartments were mostly clustered together, similar to Program I. The second major difference was that patients did not enter the community directly into one of the clustered apartments. A short-term stay at the CAP community's traditional model transitional residential program was required prior to entering the community's apartments.

This difference had several effects. First, the program could accept community members with a much higher level of current symptoms. New community members living in the transitional program could fully participate in the community, without upsetting an established apartment's status quo. The existing community members and the new members could get to know each other before making the decision to live together. At the same time, because the new person was actually a participating member of the community, it created an imperative to accept him or her into one of the apartments. As a third departure from the model, community members could also live in a non-program-run apartment in one of these same two towns and still participate in the

CAP community. In addition, this site was a bilingual and bicultural program serving both Latino and non-Latino patients.

Staff at this site were all retrained paraprofessionals from the former residential treatment program; they remained stable throughout the 4 years of the project. This program employed no patients as staff, but also had no staff turnover during the first 4 years of the project.

Program III

Program III, the suburban site, also varied from the ideal model. This program, situated in an area including some of the most expensive housing in the United States, could not locate affordable housing in large clusters. Thus, only some housing existed in small clusters; most was located in scattered sites across several suburbs. Consequently, this program did not have the advantage of proximity to foster a sense of community, and so needed to work much harder to accomplish this. Because, like Program I, this program did not have a buffer between acceptance as a new community member on the one hand, and full community membership and responsibilities as a roommate on the other, it also tended to select new community members who appeared capable of rather immediately fitting into the existing community. This tended to rule out very symptomatic new members.

The staff at this program were all initially retrained professionals from the former residential treatment program. However, in the second year of the project, the entire staff resigned, because they could not handle the changed role expectations. They were replaced by a staff of CAP community members (current "patients") and new staff without clinical or consumer experience. Because the housing in this program was more scattered, community maintenance was much more a result of staff involvement than at the other two sites. Community members had to be driven around to maintain intracommunity connections, because the suburb had a poor transportation system. This negative aspect of relying on staff for the community's maintenance was mitigated by many of the staff being community members themselves.

Program Differences

Only Program I had an independent "community center" site. Programs II and III, in areas with less available buildings, used each other's houses and staff offices for meetings and activities. This, and other factors, affected the "climate" of each community. Program I appeared less staff focused, but more chaotic and contentious. It frequently adopted social activist stances as a community, some of which were aggressively advocacy oriented and anti–treatment system. Program II, as an explicitly Latino program, had a preexisting culture for patients to fit into. Thus, as opposed to Programs I and III, it did not have to expend a large amount of time and effort creating the community's culture. Probably as a function of both preexisting culture and more involvement of professional staff from the residential treatment program, Program II appeared both more conservative and more sure of itself as a community. In Program III, perhaps because of the staff turnover midway into the project, the "personality" of that community took a longer time to assert itself. However, when it developed, especially because so many staff members were residents of the project, it had an exciting vitality of experimenting with roles and expectations.

Each program handled relationships with the treatment system slightly differently. Program II was part of a large multiprogram agency that included a CMHC model outpatient clinic. Thus, most of the Program II community members received their ongoing outpatient treatment from staff at a branch site of this outpatient clinic. Program III was a long-standing social rehabilitation agency with several residential treatment programs and a vocational rehabilitation program. However, they too created a special outpatient clinic, with separate treatment staff, initially to provide treatment services specifically to the CAP community. In both cases, this way of providing treatment did not violate the split between social and treatment supports, but having both types of support in the same agency did have the potential to infringe on this separation.

Program I was also a traditional model social rehabilitation agency originally created by families. This agency provided no specific treatment services for its CAP community members, giving them the choice of using any of the treatment system's CMHCs, ACT programs, case managers, or no treatment services at all.

Implementation of the Model and Alternatives to Hospitalization

As described in this chapter, the three CAP communities were not designed as alternatives to hospitalization per se. Their design was based on a more fundamental critique of the mental health system as a whole, rather than a critique of one aspect of the system, the hospital. Hospitalization was seen as a systematic response to repeated failures of the support system, which in most mental health systems was limited to treatment and rehabilitation supports. Many of these dependency-reinforcing treatment and rehabilitation services were seen as potentially unnecessary, or not as important, if they could be replaced by interdependent mutual supports. Because the hospital is a key component of this dependency-reinforcing treatment system, it too was seen in this light.

However, the critique of the system included hypothesized reasons for repeated hospital use by community-based patients and a structural attempt to correct this. This structural correction was the creation of permanent social supports as substitutes for treatment services functioning as supports. Consequently, it implied that then-current levels of treatment services would be unnecessary. However, each of the three CAP communities was left to develop within the broad outlines of the model, based on a self-defined response to the needs of its members.

It is significant, then, that each CAP community developed a community response for its members who were in crisis, aiming to avoid not only hospitalization, but also the use of hospital alternatives that were outside their respective CAP community. In this way, again, one can see the fundamental nature of the model's critique. The model did not critique hospitals as unnecessary, but rather aimed to place the entire treatment-rehabilitation system in what it saw as a proper role.

As mentioned earlier in this chapter, Program I reserved one of the community's apartments as a crisis apartment. A group of community members were trained to help people through crises. A community member in crisis, or a fellow community member who believed someone was experiencing a crisis, could call anyone in this group. One or more of the group would stay with the community member in crisis in the designated crisis apartment, supporting them through the emergency. Program III developed a less structured approach, believing that community members would be more comfortable being supported in their own homes. This was more of a "neighbor"-based crisis system than the more structured, professional-like system adopted by Program I.

Because the community structure in Program II was slightly different, the response to community members' crises was also different. People who experienced clinical crises stayed at the same modified residential program that they spent time at before entry to the program. The member in crisis received treatment model support throughout the crisis, without having to leave the community's more generally supportive climate.

All of the programs attempted to provide alternatives to the hospital for existing community members who experienced crises. Their goal was to avoid community disruption caused by hospitalization; therefore, use of crisis and respite alternatives to the hospital and the hospital itself was avoided. However, only Program II developed a way to act as a subacute alternative to continued stay in a hospital for new incoming community members.

The two other CAP communities, once established, were resistant to disrupt the communities' stability by bringing in new destabilized members with whom they had no preexisting relationship. Because accepting new acutely ill or subacutely ill community members would result in disruption, this presented a problem. This was seen as different from supporting an existing community member with similar levels of instability.

The third program, however, had a buffer between the hospital and full participation in the CAP community. This allowed phased participation into community life, allowed the community to become familiar with new members gradually, and provided a transitional level of professional support on the foundation of community-based mutual support. This program could then accept new members with subacute levels of need into the community after very abbreviated hospital stays. However, because of its aggressive nonhospitalization policy, what this county regarded as "subacute" was what many other places regard as acute.

Discussion

None of the communities was consistently successful in acting as an alternative to the hospital for its community members. Also, only one of the programs was partially successful in acting as an alternative to the hospital for new incoming community members. The communities were not established as hospital alternatives, but rather as non-treatment-oriented mutually supportive interdependent communities. Yet, the fact that each community developed mechanisms to avoid the hospitalization of its members and was successful some of the time points to intriguing possibilities. Thus, two questions arise: can an interdependent mutually supportive community of mental health system users act as an alternative to hospitalization, and what conditions are necessary for it to successfully do so?

Groups that see themselves as defined communities frequently attempt to provide for all the needs of their community members. This is especially true of communities that see themselves, or are seen by others, as being different from the dominant community. Therefore, it is not surprising that the CAP communities, fostered as positively defined subcultures, would also attempt to do so. Rehospitalization is a familiar event within this subculture, so it is also not surprising that the communities would choose to avoid that as one of their first community support activities.

Prerequisites for Success

Developing programs based on such a different paradigm has a far-reaching impact. Agencies, staff, patients, and mental health systems are forced to confront different assumptions and to try to establish new relationships. How this is managed by all of the parties depends on many variables that fundamentally affect outcome. However, the experience of these communities seems to indicate that the stability of the community itself is a necessary prerequisite to acting as a hospital alternative.

Community stability means several things in this context. Early in the project, CAP members shared a negatively defined subculture but had not yet become a true community. The processes of community building and developing a positive group self-image require a good deal of work, and immature communities cannot take on other major tasks during these processes. Yet, by any analysis, acting as an intended alternative to the hospital for community members is just such a major task.

However, because all three projects explicitly established hospital-alternative mechanisms very early in their history, they clearly saw this as part of their development of community and self-identity. The problem, then, was how to balance the need for unimpeded community development with projects that distract the community from its foundation-building work, but that the community believes are necessary for their identity. A stable community life may mitigate the need for rehospitalization, but consistently acting as an explicit alternative to the hospital is an overly optimistic goal during early development of the community. However, even if the community has some success in this regard, it can lead to a stronger sense of community empowerment.

The CAP experience indicates that as long as programs are not diverted from their major early task of building a stable community, starting projects such as alternatives to hospitalization can be positive. However, if the community is very unsuccessful in such projects, it can have the opposite effect. Project failure could be seen as a failure of the community itself.

Establishing the Community's Culture

A clearly defined and consistent culture that is generally accepted by community members is also important. Culture can act as a stabilizing influence on communities. Without culture, individuals must provide the stability. Whereas a certain level of this is good, overreliance on individuals for community stability has some risks. For example, the ability of an individual to act as a community stabilizer changes over time. A community that relies on a limited number of individuals to provide stability risks instability if these individuals leave or if they are no longer willing or able to act in this role.

In a sense, mutually supportive interdependent communities like CAP rely on the existence of a normal curve in the level of "functioning" of community members. Some people must always be able to provide a stabilizing personal influence, most people fall within a middle group, and thus some community members can be unstable without it disrupting the overall stability of the community itself. Communities with a strong culture can tolerate a greater level of individual instability than communities relying mostly on individuals for support.

An additional danger in relying on individuals for community stability is that the community will rely on staff when community members cannot provide stability. This carries the risk of transition from an interdependent model back to a staff-dependent model.

Host Agency Stability

Psychosocial rehabilitation agencies were used as the host organizations for the three communities. The stability and character of the host agency emerged as one of the important variables. Instability in administration invariably affects outcome in mental health programs. However, when there is stability in the professional staff, administrative instability can be mitigated. Because this professional staff buffer did not exist in the CAP communities, they were extremely sensitive to administrative instability.

These two factors of host agency stability and community culture had a considerable effect on the three CAP communities and their ability to act as hospital alternatives. Two of the communities had no preexisting cultures, and each expended a great amount of community energy to form one. Thus, the culture of these communities was in a constant state of developmental flux. This had a negative short-term effect on community stability, produced a higher level of crisis among community members, and had a negative effect on the ability of these communities to act as alternatives to the hospital for either existing or new community members. Additionally, the host agency of one of these two CAP communities was very insecure. The combination of having to establish a community culture and an insecure agency base produced a high level of instability in both the CAP community and the individual members of the community. This occurred despite having structural components that were very favorable to this community's success (e.g., housing located close together, a separate community center, and good public transportation).

On the other hand, Program II was designed to be a bicultural Latino community, and so it had a strong preexisting culture. This community still had to work out cultural details, but did not have to struggle with the big picture. Furthermore, and perhaps because it had a strong established culture, this community had an acculturation process for incoming community members. This ensured continuity in the community and allowed a phased transition into the community by new members.

This phased transition was accomplished by placing a residential treatment model program within the CAP community for exclusive use by CAP community members. This initially appeared to be a major violation of the model, but ultimately it seemed to be a component of this program's success. Perhaps this can be explained by its hybrid nature. Because it was a model from the familiar treatment system, but was within the new CAP community, it had the advantage of both worlds. This component was also used by Program II as its crisis alternative to the hospital for existing community members. Its success may indicate that patients who lived in a treatment culture for many years, but were now living in a mutual support culture, may be more secure in receiving crisis support in a treatment model program within their own CAP community.

Vehicles for Organizing Community

The vehicles used for community development appear to be a crucial variable. Program I, and to a more limited extent Program II, were able to use proximity to foster this. Program II had the additional advantage of an explicitly shared culture to assist in community development. All three programs attempted to develop the notion of a shared subculture among mental health services consumers and to use this as a positive vehicle for community development. It became clear, especially in Program III's struggles in not having proximity to rely on, that some type of strong community magnet is necessary for this model to be successful.

Conclusion

To date, the results of the CAPs acting as hospital alternatives have been equivocal. Each of the communities was able to intervene in the crises of some existing community members that, if they had not, would have inevitably resulted in hospitalization. However, none of the projects was consistently successful in doing so. This seemed partly a result of the instability inherent in a beginning community development project. The fact that the communities intervened successfully some of the time suggests that at a more established stage in the development of the communities they could be expected to be more successful more often. Thus, in addition to indications that people in a stable support system have fewer crises, it seems evident that a stable and familiar community has the potential to obviate the need for some hospitalizations for its members who have crises. This is obviously desirable at whatever level it is successful.

Rehospitalization appears to be based in part on the response pattern of both patients and professionals to situational and clinical crises among patients. Any success in having interdependent mutual support intervene first in these crises, instead of the treatment-rehabilitation system, is also desirable. The treatment-rehabilitation system resources should then be available if the interdependent social support mechanisms fail. This type of system is less disruptive to the community tenure of patients, depends less on professionals for services, and thus is more effective in human and cost considerations.

That one of the programs was able to act as a subacute alternative after short-term hospitalization for new community members is also intriguing. Because this was accomplished through developing a traditional residential treatment program as a first step to CAP community involvement, questions arise as to whether interdependent patient communities can be successful mimicking professional treatment models. Although there is some indication that success is possible in some areas like case management (Nikkel et al. 1992; Sherman and Porter 1991), counseling (McGill and Patterson 1990), and advocacy, more research needs to be done about its success and desirability with treatment and rehabilitation models, including alternatives to hospitalization.

The potential strength of this approach is, perhaps, best illustrated by an example. One of the three host agencies of the CAPs could not survive its administrative instability. This had a profound destabilizing effect on the CAP community of this agency. They were concerned about the survival of their community. However, because they had become empowered in their own community-building process, they had also become involved in the administrative decisions of the agency.

One of the leaders of this CAP community went into a severe crisis, which in any system would have led to hospitalization. Because of the turmoil in his community, they were not able to intervene in his crisis. However, another CAP community intervened and took this community member into their hospital alternative program. Because all three CAP communities had worked hard to cooperate with each other, this person was very familiar and comfortable with the other CAP community. Hospitalization was avoided, and this person returned to his own community to continue as an important community member.

I wish I could report that the communities had solid and consistent success as alternatives to hospitalization, but the success that they did have points to the need for additional research. The experiences of the CAP communities strongly indicate that interdependent mutually supportive communities could provide a more stable and satisfying community life. Ultimately, this is the best alternative to hospitalization.

References

Anthony WA, Cohen M, Farkas M, et al: Case management—more than a response to a dysfunctional system. Community Ment Health J 24:219–228, 1988

Berkman LF, Syme SL: Social networks, host resistance, and mortality: a nine-year follow-up study of Alameda County residents. Am J Epidemiol 109:186–204, 1979

Cohen CI, Sokolovsky J: Schizophrenia and social networks: ex-patients in the inner city. Schizophr Bull 4:546–560, 1978

Cohen S, Syme SL (eds): Social Support and Health. Orlando, FL, Academic Press, 1985

Dincin J, Witheridge TF: Psychiatric rehabilitation as a deterrent to recidivism. Hosp Community Psychiatry 33:645–650, 1982

Estroff SE: Making It Crazy. Berkeley, University of California Press, 1981

Fairweather GW, Sanders D, Cressler D, et al: Community Life for the Mentally Ill: An Alternative to Institutional Care. Chicago, IL, Aldine, 1969

Freddolino PP, Moxley DP, Fleishman JA: An advocacy model for people with long-term psychiatric disabilities. Hosp Community Psychiatry 11:1169–1174, 1989

Hammer M, Makiesky-Barrow S, Gutwirth L: Social networks and schizophrenia. Schizophr Bull 4:522–545, 1978

Harris M, Bergman HC: Case management and continuity of care for the "revolving-door" patient. New Dir Ment Health Serv 40:57–62, 1988

Hogan M, Carling PJ: Normal housing: a key element of a supported housing approach for people with psychiatric disabilities. Community Ment Health J 28:215–226, 1992

Jerrell JM, Teh Wei H: Cost-effectiveness of intensive clinical and case management compared with an existing system of care. Inquiry 26:224–234, 1989

Kanter J: Clinical case management: definition, principles, components. Hosp Community Psychiatry 40:361–368, 1989

Mandiberg JM: Santa Clara County Application to the Robert Wood Johnson Foundation Mental Health Services Development Program: Clustered Apartment Program. San Jose, CA, Santa Clara County Mental Health Bureau, 1987

Mandiberg JM, Telles L: The Santa Clara County clustered apartment project. Psychosocial Rehabilitation Journal 14:21–28, 1990

Mastboom J: Forty clubhouses: models and practices. Psychosocial Rehabilitation Journal 16:9–23, 1992

McGill CW, Patterson CJ: Former patients as peer counselors on locked psychiatric inpatient units. Hosp Community Psychiatry 41:1017–1019, 1990

Mitchell RE, Trickett EJ: Social networks as mediators of social support: an analysis of the effects and determinants of social networks. Community Ment Health J 16:27–44, 1980

Moran AE, Freedman RI, Sharfstein SS: The journey of Sylvia Frumkin: a case study for policy makers. Hosp Community Psychiatry 35:887–893, 1984

Morrison RL, Bellack AS: Social functioning of schizophrenic patients: clinical and research issues. Schizophr Bull 13:715–725, 1987

Mosher LR, Menn AZ: Soteria: an alternative to hospitalization for schizophrenia. New Dir Ment Health Serv 1:73–84, 1979

Moxley DP: The Practice of Case Management. Newbury Park, CA, Sage, 1989

Nikkel RE, Smith G, Edwards D: A consumer operated case management project. Hosp Community Psychiatry 43:577–579, 1992

Parrish J: The long journey home: accomplishing the mission of the community support movement. Psychosocial Rehabilitation Journal 12:108–124, 1989

Peterson R: What are the needs of chronic mental patients?, in The Chronic Mental Patient: Problems, Solutions, and Recommendations for a Public Policy. Edited by Talbott JA. Washington, DC, American Psychiatric Association, 1978, pp 39–50

Pilisuk M, Minkler M: Supportive networks: life ties for the elderly. Journal of Social Issues 36:95–116, 1980

Randolf FL, Laux B, Carling PJ: In Search of Housing. Burlington, VT, Center for Change Through Housing and Community Support, 1987

Ridgeway P, Zipple AM: The paradigm shift in residential services: from the linear continuum to supported housing approaches. Psychosocial Rehabilitation Journal 13:11–32, 1990

Sarason BR, Sarason IG, Pierce GR (eds): Social Support: An Interactional View. New York, Wiley, 1990

Sherman PS, Porter R: Mental health consumers as case management aides. Hosp Community Psychiatry 42:494–498, 1991

Stein LI, Test MA: An alternative to mental hospital treatment, I: conceptual model, treatment program, and clinical evaluation. Arch Gen Psychiatry 37:392–397, 1980

Stein LI, Test MA (eds): The training in community living model: a decade of experience. New Dir Ment Health Serv 26:1–93, 1985

Stroul BE: Community Support Systems for Persons With Long-Term Mental Illness: Questions and Answers. Rockville, MD, National Institute of Mental Health, 1988

Telles L: The clustered apartment project: a conceptually coherent supported housing program. New Dir Ment Health Serv 56:53–64, 1992

Turner JC, Shifren I: Community support systems: how comprehensive? New Dir Ment Health Serv 2:1–14, 1979

Turner JC, TenHoor WJ: The NIMH community support program: pilot approaches to needed social reform. Schizophr Bull 4:319–348, 1978

Chapter 12

Treating Acutely Psychotic Patients in Private Homes

Editor's Note

THIS CHAPTER DESCRIBES A SYSTEM OF FAMILY SPONSOR HOMES operated by the Southwest Denver Community Mental Health Center in Colorado during the 1970s and 1980s. Family sponsor homes, a network of private homes in which patients were helped through their crises by carefully screened and selected families, helped reduce the annual use of hospital beds to one per 100,000 population in southwest Denver when the system was in operation. Southwest Denver Mental Health Center no longer exists as an independent agency, and the system of family sponsor homes is not in operation. The system became a model for other agencies, however. This chapter is interesting because it describes the crisis intervention theory on which the original concept was based and indicates how rapid tranquilization was used in the management of acutely psychotic patients in these settings. This chapter and the one that follows (which describes a similar program currently in operation in Madison, Wisconsin) will be of value to those who are interested in developing a truly noninstitutional approach to acute care.

Treating Acutely Psychotic Patients in Private Homes

Paul R. Polak, M.D.
Michael W. Kirby, Ph.D.
Walter S. Deitchman, M.S.W.

Southwest Denver Community Mental Health Center (CMHC) provides one practical working model for a comprehensive system of alternatives for both acutely and chronically disabled psychiatric patients. The system has virtually supplanted the psychiatric hospital for all adult patients from southwest Denver who are treated by public mental health services. Between 1973 and 1978, Southwest Denver CMHC used an average of one hospital bed per year for the entire catchment area of 100,000 persons, in contrast to 1974–1975 averages of 43 beds and 90 beds for Colorado and the United States, respectively.

The Catchment Area

The population of the southwest Denver catchment area lives in approximately 14 district neighborhoods. These neighborhoods range from designated poverty areas to newer, fairly affluent areas. Most residents are lower-middle class, with a strong intact family orientation. Only 10% of all households are one-person households. Ethnically, the percentage of Spanish-surnamed people has increased dramatically, from 6% of the total population in 1960 to 27% in 1975.

The following chapter was originally published, in a longer form, in "Treating Acutely Psychotic Patients in Private Homes." New Directions for Mental Health Services 1:49–64, 1979. It is reproduced here with permission. This version, with a new postscript, was prepared by Paul Polak.

Antecedents of the Southwest Denver System

The southwest Denver system was strongly influenced by the results of earlier clinical research and by treatment models developed both at Dingleton Hospital in Scotland and at the Fort Logan Mental Health Center in Colorado (Polak and Jones 1973).

The Crisis of Admission

At the point of admission to the acute psychiatric ward at Dingleton Hospital in the Scottish borders, we regularly asked the patient, the patient's family, and the referring physician what each of them saw as the reason for the patient's admission to the hospital. We found that

1. Social forces were more important determinants of the patient's admission to the hospital than psychiatric symptoms.
2. A crisis of admission involving the patient and his primary living group was a regular part of the social process leading to admission (Polak 1968).
3. The crisis of admission and the patient's development or worsening of symptoms were usually the last in a series of unresolved social-systems crises, with each unresolved crisis contributing to the next.
4. Intervention in the social-systems crisis leading to admission was more important for effective treatment and posthospital adjustment than treatment procedures within the hospital. We used therapeutic community principles to work with social systems outside the hospital.

Each of these factors proved to be just as important in the United States as they had been in Scotland.

Social-Systems Intervention

The opening of the crisis division at Fort Logan Mental Health Center, the state hospital in Denver, Colorado, afforded an opportunity to examine in more detail the immediate social environment of more than 2,000 patients at the point of admission. Social-systems intervention increasingly became the primary focus for treatment activities (Polak 1971b).

The Crisis Hostel

The increased use of social-systems work in the patient's real-life setting led to decreased use of the hospital for therapeutic community work. We began to use the hospital more as a brief asylum for situations in which temporary separation between the patient and his or her family seemed constructive.

Eventually, we closed the crisis division's inpatient service for an experimental period of 6 months. During this time, we admitted patients to a house owned by a nurse who was assisted by a group of friends living in the immediate neighborhood. This crisis hostel proved to be a viable model as an inpatient alternative setting (Brook 1976). However, acutely ill patients experiencing social-systems crises need a clearly defined preexisting social structure that they can more easily enter, identify with, and leave than was provided by this informal neighborhood setting. Finally, we found that our staff were more reluctant to use psychotropic medication in a nonhospital setting, so there was less improvement in psychiatric symptoms. In the southwest Denver model, these deficiencies were corrected by using the strong preexisting social structure of healthy families and instituting a rapid tranquilization procedure in the family sponsor homes.

Southwest Denver Comprehensive System

In 1971, the Southwest Denver Community Board, an active citizens' group, was ready to hire its first director. Because no mental health center had previously existed in the area, we could design the center's mental health services to incorporate procedures for intervening in the social environment of the patient and to develop alternatives to hospitalization. A redeployment initiative moved the funding and the jobs involved in the state hospital function from Fort Logan to the mental health center, and the center took over the responsibility of providing both state hospital and CMHC services.

Crisis and Social-Systems Intervention

The crisis of admission was used as a natural entry point for social-systems intervention procedures for all adults admitted into treatment. Staff members were trained to work in the patients' homes instead of in offices, to routinely assess which social systems were producing problems in relation to the entry of a patient into treatment, and to carry out social-systems intervention procedures simultaneously with treatment procedures for individual patients.

Elimination of Staff Offices

The single most effective mechanism facilitating home visits was neither the institution of training programs nor our philosophical commitment to the concept of home visits, but rather the elimination of clinical staff offices. Instead of offices, clinicians at Southwest Denver CMHC used small soundproof cubicles that met their need for private space for filing, paperwork, and telephone calls. Conference rooms were used for clinical conferences when meeting in the patient's home was contraindicated.

Community Control

The Southwest Denver CMHC had a citizens' board that was governing, not advisory. Treating psychotic patients in residential community settings was vigorously debated by the board before approval. Since the success of the initial program, the board's enthusiastic support of the community alternative system has been crucial to its success. Board members have recruited home sponsors and volunteers and have been integral participants in the political and funding process for the community-care system.

Family Sponsor Homes

Although techniques such as crisis and social-systems intervention enabled us to treat at home the majority of patients who otherwise might have been hospitalized, we believe that keeping a patient in the real-life setting at all costs can sometimes be destructive. When temporary or permanent separation is indicated, we place the patient in a private home. This network of private homes is an innovative alternative to hospitalization. A longitudinal research study has shown that treatment in these homes is more effective, particularly from the patient's point of view, than treatment in a psychiatric hospital (Polak and Kirby 1976). The majority of psychotic patients who are hospitalized have acute problems of 1 to 2 weeks' duration, and their brief length of stay does not foster the development of a therapeutic community. Accordingly, in 1972, the center contracted with six carefully screened and selected families in southwest Denver to form the basis of our community-based intensive care system.

Each family accepted up to two patients at one time for a base fee of $7.50 per day for room, board, and patient care. Each family had a staff coordinator who was responsible for family supervision and support. Home sponsors met regularly to learn from each other and from the staff. The clinical staff member following the patient visited the home daily to conduct sessions with the patient, involving relevant members of the patient's social system. As a substitute for the 24-hour nursing rotation on a hospital ward, our psychiatric nurses used a bellboy-paging system to provide 24-hour nursing coverage to all the community treatment settings. They, in turn, were backed up by a psychiatrist on call 24 hours a day. Care was taken to ensure that a variety of family environments was available and that staff members selected the specific family that most closely matched each patient's needs.

Some family sponsors participated in formal treatment sessions; others did not. Patients participated in family chores and activities. Meaningful personal relationships often developed between family sponsors and patients, and patients frequently visited family sponsors long after formal treatment had been terminated.

The decision to remove a patient from his natural living situation was based on an evaluation of the individual and on system resources and liabilities in the context of the following four guidelines:

1. Temporary separation is indicated in the presence of an imminent and serious threat to the life of self or others, if the natural social system or other resources are insufficient to support and handle the problem of impulse control.
2. Temporary separation is indicated to provide rest and respite in some instances in which an acute crisis has overwhelmed the resources of the natural support systems. For example, a 5-day admission for rapid tranquilization in our intensive observation apartment may be indicated for an acutely psychotic young man who has stayed up all night with his family for the last 4 days.
3. Temporary placement may be indicated to provide a supportive emotional climate for isolated, lonely, and withdrawn people es-

sentially without natural social resources, so that they can develop the trust and coping ability needed to construct their own natural support system.

4. Temporary and perhaps permanent separation may be needed to break up extremely dysfunctional relationships in which the potential for changing those relationships for the better is minimal or absent. In this situation, there is a careful cost/benefit examination of the probable consequences of separation versus no separation. For example, we have seen several examples of sons, ages 20 to 30 years, living with their mothers under quite pathologically symbiotic conditions in which episodes of rage and upheaval of lethal proportions alternate with quiet periods. After provision of substitute emotional resources for the mother, the son is often a candidate for permanent removal.

After the decision of separation was made, the patient was placed in the home setting that most suitably matched his or her needs. To meet the wide range of patient needs, a diversity of environments was essential. For example, the southwest Denver system included 1) settings employing Chicano sponsors for patients for whom a Spanish-speaking Chicano cultural setting was important; 2) settings with an emphasis on nurturing, meeting dependency needs, and high levels of support; 3) settings conveying an atmosphere of practical goal setting and achievements; and 4) settings where the patient was expected to run his or her life with minimal sponsor support and input.

The role of the home sponsors highlights some of the advantages when carefully selected individuals without formal training take on responsibilities usually carried out by professional staff. The family sponsors tended quite naturally to treat patients in their homes as guests. They oriented themselves more to the strengths and positive features of patients than to their pathology, and they were much less likely than mental health professionals to view all patient behavior in an illness framework. Home sponsors were warm, outgoing, healthy people, who were rich in life experience. We provided little formal mental health training, but focused on encouraging sponsor families to use their already existing skills.

We believe that this system of small, specific, community-based social environments had a number of advantages over psychiatric hospitals:

- A number of specifically different community environments provides a more individually tailored and responsive system than the larger, less diversified environment of the psychiatric hospital.
- Sponsor families provide a clear model of healthy individual and family behavior that can be generalized to the patient's real-life setting more easily than the learning that takes place in the artificial psychiatric hospital environment.
- In this "medium is the message" age, admission to a normal home rather than a hospital makes an immediate, clear statement to the patient and his or her family. The patient is expected to have higher self-esteem, feel less stigma, and assume greater responsibility for his or her own behavior than if he or she were hospitalized.

Court Commitment Procedures

The center was designated by the state mental health authority as an official agency to perform 72-hour court-ordered evaluations and to receive court commitments. This designation was significant, because it meant that patients under court orders were ordered into treatment with the mental health center, but did not necessarily have to go to a hospital. Depending on the patient's and the family's specific needs, the patient may have been admitted directly to a family sponsor setting, or the patient may have been admitted to an inpatient setting for a brief time before going to a family sponsor home. Through a cooperative arrangement with the Denver courts, the center was contacted early in the process of commitment; as a result, patients who might otherwise have been committed on an involuntary basis could be evaluated and, if appropriate, admitted on a voluntary basis.

Psychotropic Medication

In current psychiatric practice, acutely ill schizophrenic patients are consistently undermedicated, and chronically ill schizophrenic patients are consistently overmedicated. Without the very strong emphasis on the appropriate use of psychotropic medication, the need for hospitalization in southwest Denver would triple.

The specific procedure of rapid tranquilization, which is an important component of total community care for acutely psychotic patients, has been described elsewhere (Polak 1971a). By titrating hourly doses of one or more phenothiazines against the patient's specific target symptoms of psychosis, an initial end point of significant attenuation of psychosis is reached in 4 to 6 hours. Although sleepiness may interfere with psychotherapy for the first 2 days, side effects are usually rapidly reduced on the third day, and the patient typically is much more in touch with his or her own and his or her family's problems. Our experience is that the incidence of hypotension and other side effects is much lower if the medication is administered orally. Rapid tranquilization facilitates early crisis intervention and direct social-systems intervention.

The continuous monitoring of side effects and the elicitation of vital signs before each dose by a well-trained nursing staff are essential in successful initial high–loading dose approaches to the use of psychotropic medications.

Medical Services

At Southwest Denver CMHC, there were 1.8 full-time equivalent (FTE) psychiatrists and 11 FTE nurses. Nurses were available at all times for initial evaluations of medication side effects. When patients were admitted to a family sponsor home, a psychiatrist conducted a psychiatric evaluation and a physical examination. The nurses took blood and urine specimens, which were sent to a laboratory for analysis. In all residential settings, physicians and nurses made regular rounds.

Clinical Treatment Approaches

For patients who would normally be admitted to an acute psychiatric ward for a brief period, the southwest Denver system's emphasis on crisis responsiveness, social-systems treatment, and psychotropic medication often resulted in effective treatment at home. When brief separation from the real-life setting was the most constructive option for the patient and his or her family, admission to one of the family sponsor homes was the treatment of choice.

Case Example

A 28-year-old man was referred for hospitalization because he had been hearing voices and hallucinating a smell that he identified as the smell of death. A home visit revealed that the patient had been living in a homosexual marriage for the past 2 years. Recent sexual difficulties precipitated a separation crisis, and the threat of separation was the main precipitant of the patient's acutely schizophrenic symptoms. This crisis brought up a previously unresolved separation crisis when the patient's mother died 2 years ago; the mother had some personal characteristics similar to those of the current homosexual partner. The "smell of death" represented both the possible death of the patient's current relationship and the actual death of his mother.

Because he and his partner had very little sleep for 3 days, the patient was admitted to one of the family sponsor homes. An initial loading dose of 800 mg/day of chlorpromazine orally in four divided doses was combined with marital counseling for the patient and his homosexual partner. The patient was discharged from the family sponsor home after 1 week and was placed on a maintenance dose of 300 mg/day of chlorpromazine. Marital counseling for the patient and his partner continued on a less-frequent basis in aftercare. The same clinician who participated in evaluating the initial request for service remained the main case coordinator for the duration of treatment and was responsible both for carrying out marital counseling procedures and for monitoring the effects of medication under the supervision of the psychiatrist.

Basic Principles Useful in Implementing Hospital Alternatives

The mental health system must place first priority on effective treatment of the seriously disabled psychiatric patient. The most difficult part of placing a high priority on one group of patients is deciding which other groups should be neglected in order to carry it out. In the southwest Denver system, we decided to neglect both primary prevention and the long-term outpatient treatment of patients with neurotic problems.

Hospital alternatives require effective political strategies in order to survive. For example, shifting staff jobs from hospitals to community settings requires strategies that soften the economic and political consequences of the shift.

Effective systems for the rapid administration of appropriate psychotropic medications, medical backup, and the provision of 24-hour individual and social-systems crisis intervention services are all essential for the effective operation of alternatives to acute psychiatric hospitalization. The hospital alternative you are looking for may already exist in the community you serve. Our consistent experience is that an amazing variety of social environments exists in almost every community. Many of these environments, like the family sponsor homes in southwest Denver, have previous experience with caring for handicapped individuals and respond quite favorably to the prospect of working within a contractual relationship with a mental health agency, which is often cheaper and more effective than implementing a staff-run hospital alternative setting.

Summary

In this chapter, I have attempted to provide an overview of the system of alternatives to acute psychiatric hospitalization in the southwest Denver treatment model. This system has reduced the average annual use of hospital beds in southwest Denver, a catchment area of 100,000 persons, to one bed. The essential components of Southwest Denver CMHC's system were 1) a focus on social systems and crisis intervention, 2) an organizational structure that emphasized home visits, 3) an inpatient-alternative system that utilized a network of private homes in the community for brief placement of acutely psychotic patients, and 4) a carefully monitored set of medication policies and procedures.

Postscript

The family sponsor program in southwest Denver was discontinued in 1989. In light of the basic principles for alternatives to psychiatric hospitals outlined in the above chapter, the events that led to the closing are revealing. I had been executive director for 10 years and left on friendly terms in 1981 to pursue other interests. Over the next 6 years, five executive directors were hired, at least two of whom left on unfriendly terms. This instability at the top was compounded by a lower priority on hospital alternatives by the clinical leadership. As staff turnover increased, fewer staff members were available who knew how to treat acutely ill patients and their social-systems crises without hospitalization. The family sponsor homes were increasingly used to warehouse patients, and hospitalization rates soared.

Finally, in keeping with a move to consolidate mental health services in Denver, Southwest Denver CMHC was absorbed into the larger Denver Mental Health Corporation. Shortly afterward, the family sponsors were notified that their services were no longer needed. The family sponsors sued the corporation to coerce them into honoring their contract and settled for a lump sum.

It is quite clear that alternatives to acute psychiatric hospitalization cannot survive without continued commitment to the concept by the leadership of the mental health structure in which they operate and both commitment and skill on the part of the clinical staff.

References

Brook BD, Kirby MW, Polak PR, et al: Crisis hostel: an alternative to the acute psychiatric ward, in Emergency and Disaster Management: A Mental Health Source Book. Edited by Parad HJ, Resnik HLP, Parad LG. Bowie, MD, Charles Press, 1976, pp 67–73

Polak P: The crisis of admission. Soc Psychiatry 2:150–158, 1968

Polak P: Rapid tranquilization. Am J Psychiatry 128:640–643, 1971a

Polak P: Social systems intervention. Arch Gen Psychiatry 25:110–117, 1971b

Polak P, Jones M: The psychiatric non-hospital: a model for change. Community Ment Health J 9:123–132, 1973

Polak P, Kirby MW: A model to replace psychiatric hospitals. J Nerv Ment Dis 162:13–22, 1976

Chapter 13

The Crisis Home Program of Dane County

Editor's Note

A SYSTEM OF FAMILY CRISIS HOMES BASED ON THE SOUTHWEST Denver model described in the previous chapter is in operation at Dane County Mental Health Center in Madison, Wisconsin. Six family homes provide care to a wide variety of people in crisis, most of whom would otherwise have spent time in a hospital. Many of these patients have acutely psychotic illness, and some are acutely suicidal. Violence and safety are almost never a problem—in part, because of careful selection of appropriate patients and, in part, because patients feel honored to be invited into another person's home; they try to behave with the courtesy of houseguests. For this reason, people with difficult personality disorders behave better in the crisis home than they would in a hospital ward. Like many of the programs in this book, crisis homes induce the patient to exercise self-control or what the moral management advocates of the last century used to term "moral restraint." This feature is one of the key strengths of human-scale domestic alternatives to hospital care.

The Crisis Home Program of Dane County

Russell Bennett, R.N.

I really liked the Crisis Home. It kept me from feeling abnormal, and helped me feel like a regular person.

The Crisis Home people were very nice . . . very caring.

Crisis Homes are a very good idea. They do just what they should, letting you ease back into society and into yourself.

*O*ur crisis home program began in 1987, when we recognized that our mental health system needed such a component. It is somewhat similar to the innovative Southwest Denver Community Mental Health Center program described in the previous chapter. The central goal of the program is to provide a safe, supportive, community-based alternative for patients who might otherwise be hospitalized. For example:

Mr. I., a young man with schizophrenia, decided to "see what it was like to be off meds," and he is now hearing voices and feeling very unsafe in his small apartment. His landlord, who is not sympathetic to Mr. I.'s recent behaviors, is threatening to evict him "the next time he gets weird."

Ms. P. is a woman with a long history of past hospitalizations and an equally long list of symptoms with various diagnoses. In recent years, the diagnosis of borderline personality disorder seems to be the one most commonly written in the extensive psychiatric records. When Ms.

P. is feeling terrible, she sees wrist-slashing and overdosing as the avenue to obtaining inpatient psychiatric treatment. After treatment, the staff tend to believe that the inpatient time resulted in little or no improvement. In some cases, even Ms. P. had to agree that the hospital "brought out the worst" in her.

Ms. L., an 18-year-old woman, was just determined to be medically stable after an overdose of aspirin. She said that she tried to overdose because she and her live-in boyfriend just ended their relationship. She appears to have some healthy coping skills, but also some impulsivity and dependency. She does not want to be admitted to the psychiatric hospital, but the medical staff are reluctant to "just let her go."

In short, we find that the crisis home can be helpful for many people in different situations. If I had to generalize, I would say that perhaps the most difficult situation is when the individual is in a manic or hypomanic state; the psychotic and grandiose elements combine with a general lack of sleep (for everyone in the home), creating an increasingly stressful and exhausting experience.

Crisis homes are homes of individuals and families in the community, not a "home" owned and staffed by the mental health system. As such, they are able to accomplish a number of things that are almost impossible in other parts of the mental health system. This is not to say that we do not need and use the hospital, but even there, we find that discharge to crisis homes is very helpful in allowing patients to return to the community much sooner.

In this chapter, I briefly describe the current program, how we got here, and why it works.

Background

The mental health system in Dane County has a strong outpatient focus, spending roughly 80% of its budget on such services; some mental health systems around the country spend that percentage on inpatient care. This commitment to outpatient options has given us a broad continuum of services, one of which is the crisis home program, a component of the larger emergency services unit (ESU).

The ESU is an interdisciplinary team consisting of emergency suicide prevention telephone staff, social workers, nurses, psychologists, and psychiatrists. The importance of having the crisis home program within the ESU cannot be overestimated; the ESU provides 24-hour support for crisis home families and patients and responds to emergencies at any time. ESU staff also function as gatekeepers to the inpatient system for many patients, and they are in a unique position to consider whether a crisis home is an alternative.

Program Description

There are currently six crisis homes in the program; in the past, we have been able to maintain a much smaller but effective program with as few as two homes. We generally found these provider families through advertisements in the local newspaper, although some came to the program through other means. They are certified as short-term adult foster homes and are paid $50 per day when patients are actually in the home. These people provide a bedroom, meals, a tremendous amount of empathy, and a wide array of other types of support, including medication monitoring, teaching basic living skills, and transportation. They are in close contact with the clinicians at the ESU, and these families have been quite helpful in providing us with information to help us better understand the patient. Generally, only one patient at a time is in the home.

The following facts help to clarify how this program is used. Approximately 40% of the admissions are an alternative to hospital admission, 40% are facilitated by earlier transition out of the hospital, and 20% result from a type of housing issue or "precrisis" intervention.

In 1992, we had 140 separate crisis home admissions, for a total of 443 days of crisis home time. The average length of stay was only 3 days (see "Setting Up a Crisis Home Admission" section for further discussion). Approximately 70% of the patients are on disability income, such as Supplemental Security Income (SSI) or Social Security Disability Income (SSDI), and have symptoms diagnosed as a major mental illness, such as schizophrenia, bipolar disorder, or depression. Therefore, we can bill Medicare or Medicaid for much of the clinical time used to facilitate and maintain a crisis home admission (although the actual payment to home providers is not billable and is paid for by Dane County Mental Health Center).

Many patients have symptoms with a primary or secondary diagnosis of a character disorder. Perhaps surprisingly, people with symptoms diagnosed as borderline personality disorder have not been unusually challenging guests for the crisis home families. This topic could be the focus of an entire book, but, for now, we can say simply that the normalizing home environment, combined with a high degree of individual attention, appears to enhance any coping skills the patient may have. In our experience, this has contrasted sharply with the types of behavior we have seen in the same patients during inpatient care.

Setting Up a Crisis Home Admission

We never force patients to use a crisis home; if, after we explain the concept to them, they are adamantly against this option, we still may try to encourage them to at least "give it a try." A skeptical patient will sometimes agree, if given enough details about the home and family (e.g., where it is, what it looks like, the name of the family dog). On occasion, we even have a patient visit a home first or talk to the provider on the telephone. Many patients who are initially very resistant begin to greatly appreciate the crisis home option.

If a patient is at least willing to give it a try, we complete the necessary paperwork, which consists of an assessment of risk factors, a brief treatment plan, a signed agreement with the patient, and a copy of the crisis home guidelines for the patient. Based on the above information, we call a home provider who seems to match the specific patient's requests and needs. We explain the situation on the telephone, and, if the family is willing to have this patient in their home, we set up a time to bring the patient over. At the home, we briefly make introductions, go over the plan for the stay, and then we leave. We make it very clear that the stay must be comfortable with both the patient and the home provider and that if either has questions or concerns, they can call our 24-hour crisis line.

We originally thought that we needed home providers who could provide 24-hour support. This quickly proved to be unnecessary and even inappropriate in many situations. Once patients feel safe and supported in a crisis home, they often are able to spend significant amounts of time alone, either in the home or in the community. It may take only a few minutes, or as much as a few days, for this feeling of support and safety to develop.

The home provider and the guest often appreciate daily "check-in" contact, usually by telephone, between the ESU and the crisis home. It is an opportunity for the ESU to monitor how things are going, to offer reminders to the patient, and to change the plan as necessary. It also is a psychological reminder to the home provider and guest that they are not "alone out there" and that our support and concern are real and only a telephone call away. We often have in-person contact as well, but only as needed for dealing with the sometimes numerous and overlapping problems of finances, housing, and psychiatric symptoms. Because of the recent crisis, the patient is often on a new medication or new dose; we assess how the change is working, both on the telephone and in person.

At least 50% of the crisis home patients receive mental health services from other parts of the system, and these service providers are expected to stay involved with their patient while he or she is in a crisis home.

From the description earlier in the chapter, it may seem like getting someone into a crisis home and having things go well is relatively easy. Sometimes it is; often it is not. For one thing, it takes time, especially if a patient must be driven to a crisis home that is not nearby. Sometimes a home is not available; sometimes the home provider family is unable to accept a patient—they always have the option of declining to be open for any period of time or any specific patient situation. Admission to crisis homes generally occurs between 8:00 A.M. and 10:00 P.M., so if the crisis occurs at 3:00 A.M., a safe but temporary plan is needed.

It has been remarkable, however, how often things *do* work out, home provider and guest both stating that they are pleased with the experience. Often, a patient has had such a positive experience that he or she is willing to consider (albeit reluctantly) future reduction or even elimination of the inpatient option.

For patients who have become psychologically dependent on the inpatient milieu, we offer, at times, a plan whereby the person receives 2 or 3 days per month of crisis home time; the patient is the primary decision maker as to when to use these days, reducing the likelihood of a power struggle or an attempt to "prove" to the clinician that the patient really needs help. People who use the homes in this fashion account for the average length of stay of only 3 days; factoring out this use of crisis homes, the average stay is closer to 5 days.

Some patients get to know several crisis home families and request to be with a specific crisis home family. Unless contraindicated for some reason, we try to honor those requests.

Why Does It Work?

Several positive psychological factors may have varying degrees of significance in any given crisis home admission:

- *The name itself.* The word "crisis" acknowledges feelings of hurt, need, and struggle; "home" implies a sense of belonging and safety.
- *Using private homes.* The patient often feels very honored to be a guest in someone's home. In many cases, it has been years since the patient has been in such a pleasant living situation, if ever, and it is obviously appreciated. Even the severely dysfunctional patient will rise to the occasion and do his or her absolute best to be a safe and welcome guest.
- *Nonprofessional home providers.* Just as the patient becomes a "guest" once in the home, the home providers are just "nice people." They are often immediately trusted more than professionals and tend not to get into the power struggles that might otherwise occur.

Potential Problems

I would be remiss if I did not discuss some of the problems we have encountered. Although a home provider has never been pushed or hit in a home, staff members did have one physical confrontation in the home with an intoxicated patient. More often, the problem is that, for whatever reason, it just "doesn't work out." This is to be expected, given our admittedly imperfect abilities to assess the mental health needs of all people in all situations.

Other Problems

Neighborhood opposition is one problem that can be minimized by having the home provider talk with each of the neighbors individually, explaining that guests are carefully screened and to *please* let us know if there are any problems or concerns. As certified adult foster homes, no public hearing is required before a family agrees to share its home in this fashion.

There is no doubt that setting up such a program opens up a variety of liability issues. Without going into detail, our home providers are now insured through the mental health center, but, for many years, each provider had to obtain insurance from their own agencies. It is critical that everyone involved in the program acknowledge the risks, perhaps even valuing these risks as necessary and positive elements of any quality human life (and any quality mental health system).

Tragedies are another problem; for example, several suicidal patients did kill themselves in the days or weeks after staying at crisis homes. Other tragedies have also occurred. This has proven to be very difficult for our home providers, but to my knowledge, none has left the program for this reason. In such situations, the home providers have joined involved professionals and family members in processing the impact of such a loss.

Summary

For those who are interested in learning more about the crisis home concept, I recommend reading *Crisis Residential Services in a Community Support System,* an excellent overview by Beth Stroul, available through the National Institute of Mental Health. I welcome questions, as do our crisis home providers and emergency services staff.

Our crisis home program can never be the perfect option for every mental health crisis; we will continue to use the hospital for those who need it. Nonetheless, the crisis home is the choice for many people in many different situations, offering many advantages over the hospital, not the least of which is how the patient begins to think of himself or herself and the illness. To be truly welcomed into a home is something we all deserve to experience.

For me, what I see and hear from the people directly involved is the ultimate proof that what we offer is working. Our first crisis home family from 6 years ago is still in the program; I encourage you to read her words later in this chapter, in "Finding Crisis Home Families."

In an exit survey, 90% of the patients were glad to have the option of going to a crisis home. Having a "time out from a stressful situation" was most often identified as what was helpful to them, as was "being treated like a normal person." In the words of one guest:

> Being in an environment where support and safety could be obtained outside the sterile walls of the hospital is always the better alternative. The crisis home family did more for me than any hospital could have ever offered me.

Finding Crisis Home Families

As a national training site for outpatient mental health services, the Dane County Mental Health Center has many visitors every year. I often discuss the crisis home program with these visitors and try to take them to one of our crisis homes to meet with a provider family (and any guest who is in the home and chooses to participate). During such visits, a number of questions are generated.

What motivates an individual or family to become a crisis home provider?   The motivations seem to be as individual as the providers themselves. Some are young families in which one of the parents needs to be home most of the time anyway. Others are people who already have raised a family and have extra room and time. Some have financial considerations and can use $50 a day. I have no problem with that; but none of our home providers is in it just for the money. All of our home providers appear to share some sense of individual responsibility for helping others. Some have a strong sense of religious or spiritual conviction, although none has ever attempted to proselytize.

What are you looking for in a home provider?   You do not need to be an expert in mental health to be a crisis home provider, although you may become one. We train and teach about mental illness, and support and information are available to the providers 24 hours a day. Far more important is that they have certain interpersonal skills:

- To be able to welcome someone into their home without being tense or "fake"
- To be able to acknowledge the problems of the patient without feeling obligated to try to solve such problems
- To know when they need to call us for advice or some type of intervention
- To recognize and hopefully draw out the strengths of even the most severely disabled guests in their home

Each home provider is unique and has a "style" for doing this type of work. In May 1987, Krista Roys and her family became our first crisis home provider; the skills and "style" of her family have been essential elements in shaping the program as it exists today. This chapter concludes with some of Krista Roys' thoughts, which reflect the spirit of the program and the interpersonal skills I am always delighted to see in a potential crisis home provider.

> When my family and I took the plunge to become a crisis home for Dane County Mental Health Center, I wondered if we (not our guests) could be "normal" enough for the job. Could we seem as balanced as the Huxtables while carrying on our family life before a live audience? How would it be to have a stranger showering in my bathroom who would also partake in the chaos that sometimes passes for domesticity in the kitchen? And, more importantly, would we be "good for" the people who would come to our home as guests?
>
> Now that we have weathered 6 years together, I have tentative answers. Concerns about appearances long ago gave way to the inescapable yet comfortable truth that we can't stay dressed-up for long at our house. If mom and the kids are skirmishing over dirty socks in the corner or are engaged in a lively discussion about the merits of practicing this week's least favorite piano tune—well, welcome to our world. Sometimes these struggles even dissolve more quickly if we're lucky enough to have another person with a fresh outlook in our midst. A houseguest can throw a little light on some of our standard operating procedures.
>
> Somehow our guests have not stayed strangers for long. With the kaleidoscope of personalities who have come to stay with us, I'm struck by the fact that overwhelmingly we have enjoyed their presence. Yes, there is fragility, awkwardness at times, and wrenching pain that also touches our family in surprising ways. But our guests have been so accepting of us and our fragility, that, far from feeling invaded by people with "problems" it's more as though our family enlarges a little at intervals.
>
> Finally, it turns out that, in spite of ourselves, we often are "good for" the person staying with us. As it is for everyone, there are days when a lot happens in our family; we have a lot of chores to tackle, a lot of turmoil to handle in our own lives. There's not always time to consciously channel energy into the role of helper for someone else. Though we acknowledge the emotional challenge facing our guest, it's almost as if circumstances conspire to leave the "disorder" behind for periods in the day; taking such a break seems to fortify the person. It is clear to me that often I have ended up on the *receiving* end of the helping that happens here; this has been the lesson most useful to me about living in a crisis home.

From Patient Management to Risk Management

Richard Warner, M.B., D.P.M.

*M*any may wonder whether the human-scale programs described in this book—nearly all of them unlocked, domestic, and informal in style—can address the needs of the difficult-to-treat patients who form a core constituency for community mental health care systems. Can these programs handle patients who are violent or on criminal charges, patients who actively resist treatment, patients with acquired immunodeficiency syndrome (AIDS) or other medical problems, patients who prefer to live on the streets, and patients who combine substance use with mental illness? The table below, which presents information compiled from the authors of the previous chapters, reveals that North American programs that are integrated with or contract with a broader community treatment system clearly do not exclude such patients.

In most of these programs, patients who have committed misdemeanors and, often, felonies are routinely accepted into treatment. In some instances, as at Cedar House in Boulder, Colorado, offenders are transferred directly from jail into treatment, after evaluation by an outreach team. Similarly, outreach workers locate mentally ill homeless people at the local shelter; these people may then be admitted to an alternative facility, involuntarily if necessary. A large proportion of the patients at Crossing Place in Washington, D.C., are homeless; an outreach team invites homeless mentally ill people to visit the house, and, sometimes, after many attempts, some agree to stay. Few people are discharged from these alternative programs without first establishing a reasonable living situation.

Agitation and disruptiveness, threatening behavior, or imminent risk of violence or self-harm are not usually grounds for exclusion. In

Madison, Wisconsin, agitated patients who are imminently suicidal may be placed in private family homes, as they were in the similar family sponsor home program in southwest Denver while it was in operation. All of the alternative programs that are affiliated with a mental health system accept AIDS patients, and a few programs admit patients with significant medical problems that require nursing care, such as brittle diabetes, leg ulcers that require daily dressing, illnesses that require patients to use oxygen, and indwelling urinary catheters. These programs also often accept patients with acute organic confusional states in order to pursue the diagnosis of the medical cause of the condition.

Lack of cooperation with treatment does not exclude patients from an alternative treatment setting. Virtually all of the programs accept people who are at risk of walking away from treatment, and most accept patients who are detained under involuntary treatment orders when allowed by the state statute. Northwest Evaluation and Treatment Center in Seattle, a locked setting that admits only involuntary patients,

Characteristics of 13 hospital alternative programs

	CH	V	CP	PF	NE
Inpatient capacity	15	20	8	8–10 per house	32
Carry outpatients?	6	Evaluations	Sometimes	No	No
Associated with community mental health system:					
as an integral part	Yes	Yes	No	Yes	Yes
by contractual agreement	—	—	Yes	—	—
Cost/patient/day	$160	$160	$156	$215–$230	$249
Cost as % of private hospital cost	25	36	17	33	31
Cost as % of state hospital cost	57	54	35	66	83

Note. CH = Cedar House, Boulder; V = Venture, Vancouver; CP = Crossing Place, Washington, D.C.; PF = Progress Foundation, San Francisco; NE = Northwest Evaluation, Seattle.

treats many patients who are not welcome at local private hospitals.

The severity of illness of patients in these alternatives is apparent from the case descriptions in many of the chapters. At Burch House, a psychotic Vietnam veteran crawls around on his belly and stays up all night on guard against the enemy. In the Windhorse program, a patient mutters and snarls to himself continually and has periods of agitation and destructiveness. A catatonic patient at Cedar House is near mute, almost immobile, and scarcely eats or drinks. Recent comparative research (Warner and Huxley 1993) documents the high degree of pathology at one of these alternatives. A sample of patients at Cedar House was shown, on a standardized measure, to be significantly more disturbed than long-term patients on the ward of a district general hospital in Manchester, England. Cedar House patients had higher levels of both positive symptoms of psychosis and affective symptoms. Despite the greater severity of illness, the quality of life (measured by a standard quality of life profile) of the Cedar House residents was significantly better than that of the hospitalized patients.

CI	SP	SB	BH	W	CA	FSH	CHs
10–12	6	8	8	1 per house	60–75 per program	2 per home in 3 homes	1 per home in 6 homes
1–10	Drop in	Informal	No	Yes	N/A	No	Informal only
Yes	No	No	No	No	Yes	Yes	Yes
—	No	Yes	No	No	—	—	—
$300–$365	$125	$300	$85	$169–$238	$12–$27	$150 (1980s)	$80
200	18	75	11	25	N/A	33	12
200	39	100	22	80	N/A	60	20 (continued)

CI = Crisis Intervention, Netherlands; SP = Soteria Project, California; SB = Soteria Berne, Switzerland; BH = Burch House, New Hampshire; W = Windhorse, Massachusetts; CA = Clustered Apartments, Santa Clara County; FSH = Family Sponsor Homes, Denver; CHs = Crisis Homes, Madison.

Characteristics of 13 hospital alternative programs *(continued)*

	CH	V	CP	PF	NE
Does program accept patients with:					
serious imminent suicide risk?	Sometimes	No	Yes	Yes	Yes
serious nonimminent suicide risk?	Yes	Yes	Yes	Yes	Yes
nonserious suicide attempts/threats?	Yes	Yes	Yes	Sometimes	Yes
agitation and disruptiveness?	Sometimes	Sometimes	Yes	Yes	Yes
imminent risk of violence?	No	No	Sometimes	Yes	Yes
current threatening/ menacing behavior?	Rarely	No	Yes	Yes	Yes
obnoxious interpersonal behavior?	Yes	Yes	Yes	Yes	Yes
organic confusional states?	Yes	No	Yes	Usually	Yes
significant medical problems (such as brittle diabetes, indwelling urinary catheter)?	Yes	Yes	No	No	No
AIDS?	Yes	Yes	Yes	Yes	Yes
significant substance use problems?	Yes	Yes	Yes	Yes	Yes
risk of drug/alcohol withdrawal reaction?	Sometimes	No	Sometimes	Yes	Yes
current drug/ alcohol intoxication?	No	No	Sometimes	Usually	Yes
involuntary treatment order/civil commitment?	Yes	No	No	No	Yes
current misdemeanor criminal proceedings?	Yes	Yes	Yes	Yes	Yes
current felony criminal proceedings?	Yes	No	Sometimes	Yes	No
risk of escape/walking away from treatment?	Sometimes	Yes	Yes	Yes	Yes

Note. CH = Cedar House, Boulder; V = Venture, Vancouver; CP = Crossing Place, Washington, D.C.; PF = Progress Foundation, San Francisco; NE = Northwest Evaluation, Seattle.

CI	SP	SB	BH	W	CA	FSH	CHs
Sometimes	Yes	Yes	No	No	Yes	Yes	Yes
Sometimes	Yes	Yes	Yes	Sometimes	Yes	Yes	Yes
Yes	Yes	Yes	Yes	Yes	Yes	No	Yes
No	Yes	Sometimes	Yes	Sometimes	Yes	Usually	Yes
No	Yes	Sometimes	Sometimes	No	Sometimes	No	No
No	Yes	Usually	Sometimes	Sometimes	Sometimes	Sometimes	No
Sometimes	Yes	Usually	Sometimes	Yes	Usually	Yes	Sometimes
No	No	No	No	Sometimes	No	Usually	Usually
No	No	No	No	Sometimes	No	Sometimes	Usually
Sometimes	N/A	No	Yes	Yes	Yes	N/A	Yes
No	Yes	No	Rarely	Usually	Sometimes	Usually	Usually
No	No	Sometimes	No	No	No	No	Sometimes
No	No	No	No	No	Sometimes	No	No
No	No	No	No	Sometimes	No	Yes	Yes
Sometimes	Yes	Sometimes	Sometimes	Yes	Yes	Yes	Yes
No	No	Sometimes	No	Yes	No	Usually	Sometimes
Yes	Yes	Yes	Sometimes	Sometimes	No	Yes	Yes

CI = Crisis Intervention, Netherlands; SP = Soteria Project, California; SB = Soteria Berne, Switzerland; BH = Burch House, New Hampshire; W = Windhorse, Massachusetts; CA = Clustered Apartments, Santa Clara County; FSH = Family Sponsor Homes, Denver; CHs = Crisis Homes, Madison.

Patient Selection

The selection of appropriate patients for the alternative settings is usually made by the crisis staff and psychiatrist of the mental health system after consultation with the staff of the acute facility. Patients who are inappropriate for admission to the alternative facility are likely to be admitted instead to a hospital, an alcohol detoxification facility, or other accommodation. In the Madison crisis home program, the program coordinator usually determines who will be admitted, but the crisis home family and the patient have veto power. In most instances (e.g., at Crossing Place, Venture, and Cedar House), the facility staff, with the backup of the house director when necessary, have the final decision about whether an admission is appropriate.

Progress Foundation in San Francisco has a virtual "no refusal" policy for its acute alternative houses. Psychiatric emergency staff at San Francisco General Hospital act as gatekeepers and select appropriate patients for admission. The patient is interviewed at the emergency room by a liaison from the Progress Foundation who makes a referral to one of the houses. The patient is automatically accepted unless, on arrival at the house, the patient's symptoms escalate and inpatient care becomes necessary. Occasionally, a patient may not be accepted if his or her condition is not sufficiently acute to require admission.

Patient Management

The broad acceptance of patients who would prove difficult even for a locked hospital unit raises the question, how are such patients managed?

How do staff react, for example, when an intoxicated patient returns to his or her residential treatment facility? In many instances, such as at Crossing Place in Washington, D.C., or Venture in Vancouver, the patient is initially handled in a low-key manner, if possible, and isolated (or sent to bed) until he or she is thinking more clearly. In Vancouver and Boulder, a grossly intoxicated or obnoxious patient may be transferred to a local detoxification facility until sober; he or she can then return to the treatment facility. At Burch House in New Hampshire, if the problem is recurrent, the therapeutic community must resolve it. At the Progress Foundation in San Francisco, repeated substance use is dealt with in an individualized way. Steve Fields, the director, reports:

For some patients, the treatment plan includes working with them despite the use of substances. Others may have reached a point at which they have a "no drinking or using" clause in their admission agreement. In those cases, the patient might be discharged to a program for patients with substance use problems. The disposition—to be hospitalized, to be discharged to another program, or to remain in the acute residential treatment program—would depend on the relative psychiatric stability of the patient.

Similarly, the response to patients who become assaultive or destructive is determined, in most programs, by clinical and diagnostic considerations—although the first consideration in all of the settings is to ensure the safety of the patient, other residents, and staff. At Venture in Vancouver, for example, if a resident in an acutely psychotic state assaults someone or damages property, the staff and psychiatrist assess the situation. An assaultive psychotic patient would probably be transferred to the hospital. If nonserious property damage occurred, the patient might be given additional medication and allowed to stay in the facility. If a patient with a personality disorder assaulted someone, the patient would probably be discharged. At Venture, Crossing Place, or Cedar House, an attempt would be made to bill the patient for damaged property, and, at some facilities, criminal charges may be brought against an assaultive or destructive patient, especially if he or she is not acutely psychotic.

In noninstitutional settings where restraints and seclusion are not used, it is important to minimize a disturbed patient's agitation as soon as possible to prevent disruption of the environment and to ensure the safety of the patient and others. On admission to Cedar House, psychotic patients are likely to be offered benzodiazepines, such as diazepam (Valium), as needed to reduce anxiety, agitation, and psychotic symptoms, in addition to standard doses of antipsychotic or mood-stabilizing medication. Agitated patients often require extra staff support and supervision to reduce anxiety and to ensure that they are not intrusive with other patients and do not walk away from the facility. Firm direction of the patient may be required, but head-to-head confrontation is avoided. A staff member or volunteer may take the patient for a walk to the park or involve him or her in another activity to help reduce tension and restlessness.

It is not uncommon for a resident, especially one with a personality disorder, in an acute care setting to make a nondangerous self-harm gesture such as a superficial cut on the arm or wrist. At most of these alternative settings (e.g., at Soteria, Burch House, and Windhorse), staff respond to these gestures by sitting and talking with the patient about what led to the behavior and by encouraging him or her to talk to the staff in the future before making such gestures. Some of the facilities, such as Crossing Place and Cedar House, emphasize that the response should be understated and not reinforce the behavior by providing more attention than is strictly necessary to ensure the patient's safety and to provide medical care. At none of the programs, except the crisis home program in Madison, would such behavior lead to the patient being discharged or transferred. Even in Madison, such patients will almost always be given a second chance to return to the crisis home, in which case the patient appears to learn from the first experience and does not repeat the self-harm behavior.

Follow-up Care

Most of the programs described in this book are integral components of a broad community care system or have a close contractual relationship with one. They generally ensure continuity of care for patients by making discharge planning an integral part of the residential treatment plan and through multiteam meetings. In Boulder, executive staff and the managers of the intensive outpatient, hospital, and Cedar House programs meet weekly to review the progress and community treatment needs of all patients receiving acute care. In Vancouver, similar multi-service meetings are held to review the treatment of patients who are proving difficult to manage, and the crisis team and the acute care facility maintain a log of treatment plans for difficult patients.

Some of the programs allow outpatient contact with the acute care facility to continue after the patient is discharged. At Venture, daily drop-in for former patients is encouraged to allow for reassessment if they are not doing well. Ex-residents of the crisis home programs in Madison and southwest Denver often visit the family care sponsors on an informal basis just to stay in touch. Ex-residents of Soteria Berne maintain contact with the treatment community while attending other agencies for outpatient care. At Crossing Place, previous residents may visit on "drop-in night;" others visit and come for dinner at different times. At Cedar House, some patients may remain at the house after discharge for a few days or weeks to receive extra supervision or monitored medicines; others may drop in for support or meals as an interim measure to prevent the necessity of admission; and many welcome the opportunity to return as outpatients for Thanksgiving and Christmas dinner.

Benefits

The flexibility of these alternative settings permits them to respond to the human needs of their clientele and, along with their nonalienating and domestic character, adds to their strengths. Patients who would otherwise be in an institutional setting can retain autonomy and maintain links to the community. People who have used the crisis home programs in Madison and Denver feel less stigmatized by the experience than by hospital admission because treatment takes place in a truly normalizing environment where contact is only with mentally healthy people. Patients at Cedar House, Progress Foundation, Crossing Place, and elsewhere maintain many of their social skills as a result of the expectation that they will perform domestic chores and continue to deal with many of their usual social responsibilities. Windhorse, which treats people in their own homes, goes furthest in empowering the patient in this respect; the patient has ownership of the household and responsibility for all household management. Virtually all patients who have used alternative facilities—over 90% of Progress Foundation patients, for example—say that they prefer the experience to the hospital.

The unusually supportive and personalized care in the nontraditional programs—at Soteria and Soteria Berne, Burch House, and Windhorse—means that psychotic patients can be treated with much lower doses of neuroleptic medication than is usual in standard inpatient care. At Soteria Berne, the doses of antipsychotic medication used are about one-quarter of those employed at hospitals in the area. The lower cost of alternative settings means that the pace of treatment is slower than in a hospital; patients can be evaluated for a longer time before drug therapy is begun, patients do not have to make a quick decision about medications, and dosages can be increased gradually.

For the mental health system, hospital alternatives offer several advantages. They permit scarce hospital beds to be reserved for other very severely disturbed patients who require intensive care. If the program is an integral component of the community agency, access for patients in need of inpatient care is ensured and is not dependent on hospital bed availability and other factors beyond the agency's authority; quality of inpatient care is under the direct control of the community agency; and integrated treatment with good continuity of care is much more readily accomplished. Hospital alternatives create an additional option for the care of patients in crisis. The crisis centers in the Netherlands provide immediate care for patients with a host of psychosocial problems that would not warrant or benefit from hospital admission. For patients with severe personality disorders who may become more out of control in a hospital, the availability of a normalizing alternative placement may be much more clinically appropriate.

Cost

An important advantage of hospital alternatives is their low cost. As the table shows, the programs that are integral to or in a close working relationship with a community care system (i.e., Cedar House, Crossing Place, Progress Foundation, Northwest Evaluation and Treatment Center, and the crisis homes in Madison and Denver) are more cost-effective than hospital care. These programs cost an average of one-quarter of the expense of local private hospital care and never more than one-third; they cost an average of a little more than one-half of the expense of state hospital care. Their small size explains much of the savings. Unlike hospitals, they do not require expensive dedicated service elements such as pharmacies, security personnel, laboratories, or emergency departments. The alternative facility often obtains the services provided by these components of a hospital from an equivalent in the community. For example, at Cedar House, the local police department provides the same function as hospital security personnel, when required, and laboratory services and medical investigations are obtained by contracts with community agencies and hospital outpatient departments.

The staffing flexibility of community mental health agencies, the use of multidisciplinary teams, and the delegation of responsibility also permit considerable cost savings. In hospitals, protocols established by the medical staff and imposed by accreditation requirements and liability concerns lead to increased staffing requirements. For example, in many good private hospitals, a reasonable caseload for a full-time psychiatrist might be about 10 inpatients; at a community alternative, however, a psychiatrist could care for this many patients in one-half the time. He or she would accomplish this by delegating to well-trained mental health professionals many of the daily evaluation and treatment tasks—individual and family psychotherapy, gathering clinical background information, and disposition planning.

Risks and Risk Management

Many mental health professionals may be concerned that open-door and more informal inpatient treatment facilities present greater risks in the care of severely disturbed patients. This need not be the case, however. Clearly, open-door facilities require careful selection of patients, day-by-day observation of the resident's changing condition, and expert supervision of treatment plans to ensure safety. The setting may be informal in style, but staff can never be casual in their efforts to observe and protect their patients. Patients are not admitted if they are at risk of walking away and if walking away is likely to lead to a serious problem. A patient who is so psychotic and agitated that he or she may run out into traffic is likely to be placed in a hospital. A resident who becomes so confused or autistic that he or she cannot follow staff direction will require additional staffing for continuous observation or transfer into a safer setting.

A key to risk management in these settings is excellent program supervision. Knowledgeable and experienced professionals must have daily input into the development of treatment plans. At some of the more medically oriented treatment facilities, such as Venture and Cedar House, psychiatrists may be an important part of this daily supervision; at the more nontraditional programs, such as Windhorse and Burch House, psychiatrists are less closely involved, but supervision by experienced professionals is equally close and detailed. The open-door environment requires a higher than usual level of staff skill and attention. More responsibility for risk prevention is delegated to staff and, to a degree, to patients—giving patients the message that they are responsible for themselves. This delegation of control and responsibility is an important reason that these facilities are less alienating than the hospital setting.

Given this degree of care and professionalism in program operation, the level of risk does not appear to be higher for these programs.

Comparative figures are not available, but anecdotal reports indicate that untoward consequences are rare and unlikely to be greater than for hospital care. In the Madison program, for example, no patient has ever assaulted a crisis home provider, although property damage and theft have occurred on occasion. Similarly, at Cedar House, aggression and assault are less common than in a hospital. It is certainly true that patients not uncommonly walk away from treatment at Cedar House and need to be brought back by family members or the police; elopement with resulting bad outcome, however, has been very rare. Over nearly 2 decades of operation, occurrences of this type, or similar critical incidents such as serious suicide attempts on premises, have been no more frequent than for the mental health center's patients placed in hospitals.

Many professionals would argue, moreover, that the greatest risk for seriously mentally ill patients is not while they are in inpatient treatment (of any type), but *after discharge,* when they may evade outpatient treatment and become severely disturbed again. If this is the case, lower-cost, less-alienating alternative facilities that are closely integrated with the outpatient system of care may reduce risk to the patients in the long run by allowing a longer period of inpatient treatment, by developing a better allegiance with patients, and by leading to the formulation of a successful community treatment plan. Those who work in community mental health are very familiar with the concept that short-term concerns about liability and risk have to be weighed against long-term benefits for the patient and overall quality of life. Nowhere is this more evident than in the choice of alternatives to hospital treatment.

Reference

Warner R, Huxley P: Psychopathology and quality of life among mentally ill patients in the community: British and US samples compared. Br J Psychiatry 163:505–509, 1993

Index

*Page numbers printed in **boldface** type refer to tables or figures.*